# MR. HUMBLE

## AND

# DR. BUTCHER

*A Monkey's Head, the Pope's Neuroscientist,*
*and the Quest to Transplant the Soul*

## BRANDY SCHILLACE

### SIMON & SCHUSTER

*New York   London   Toronto   Sydney   New Delhi*

Simon & Schuster
1230 Avenue of the Americas
New York, NY 10020

First Simon & Schuster hardcover edition March 2021

SIMON & SCHUSTER and colophon are registered trademarks of Simon & Schuster, Inc.

For information about special discounts for bulk purchases,
please contact Simon & Schuster Special Sales at 1-866-506-1949
or business@simonandschuster.com.

The Simon & Schuster Speakers Bureau can bring authors to your live event.
For more information or to book an event,
contact the Simon & Schuster Speakers Bureau
at 1-866-248-3049 or visit our website at www.simonspeakers.com.

*Interior design by Ruth Lee-Mui*

Manufactured in the United States of America

1  3  5  7  9  10  8  6  4  2

Library of Congress Cataloging-in-Publication Data
Names: Schillace, Brandy, author.  Title: Mr. Humble and Dr. Butcher : a monkey's head,
the Pope's neuroscientist, and the quest to transplant the soul / Brandy Schillace.
Description: First Simon & Schuster hardcover edition. | New York : Simon & Schuster, 2021. |
Includes bibliographical references and index.
Identifiers: LCCN 2020038727 (print) | LCCN 2020038728 (ebook) |
ISBN 9781982113773 (hardcover) | ISBN 9781982113827 (ebook)
Subjects: LCSH: White, Robert Joseph, 1926–2010. | Neurosurgeons—United States—Biography. |
Transplantation of organs, tissues, etc.—United States—History. | Medical ethics—United States—History.
Classification: LCC RD592.9.W54 A3 2021  (print) |
LCC RD592.9.W54  (ebook) | DDC 617.4/8092 [B]—dc23
LC record available at https://lccn.loc.gov/2020038727
LC ebook record available at https://lccn.loc.gov/2020038728

ISBN 978-1-9821-1377-3
ISBN 978-1-9821-1382-7 (ebook)

# Contents

## Acknowledgments

*A book like this one only comes into being through the good offices of a small army.* I wish to thank Doron Weber and the Alfred P. Sloan Foundation Program in Public Understanding of Science, Technology, and Economics for their generous research support. I also wish to thank the Hosking Houses Trust, which allowed me a month's residency to do final edits (both necessary and brutal!) without interruption. Additionally, I wish to thank the family of Dr. Robert White, especially Patty and Michael, and also Kreg Vetovitz for his help accessing materials about his father, Craig.

To Dr. Lesley Sharp and Dr. Michael DeGeorgia, my deep appreciation for your expertise throughout the project (and I owe you much whiskey, Michael, for that first introduction to the bloodstained notebook).

To Masha and the Russian Medical Museum of the FSSBI, N. A. Semashko National Research Institute of Public Health, my sincere thanks for your aid in finding materials on Vladimir Demikhov.

To the many people I interviewed, thank you for your time and your willingness.

And last but by no means least, thanks to fellow writer Lance Parkin for endless rounds of lunch discussion over drafts—and to my partner, Mark Schillace, who listened patiently as I read every single chapter out loud. Many times. Even on car trips. You are a magical unicorn.

*T*here *are times when a story finds you, and not the other way around. This one* begins with a telephone call from an old friend . . . a friend who happens to be a brain surgeon.

Dr. Michael DeGeorgia invites me to his small, square office on the campus of Cleveland's Case Western Reserve University. When I arrive, he kindly asks me to take a seat, because some stories are better told when you aren't in danger of falling over. "I'd like to show you something," he says, reaching into his bottom desk drawer.

It's a shoe box, slightly worn. He slides the unassuming package across the desk and I lift the lid with some eagerness and a touch of trepidation. "It's not a brain, is it?" I ask. No, he tells me. Or at least, *not exactly.*

A computation notebook, faded and brown and labeled Massachusetts Institute of Technology, lies on top. The name Robert J. White has been written on the front. As I turn the pages, I see cramped writing, old glue, and spots of rust here and there. "Probably mouse blood," Michael says. It's an experimental record. I hold in my hands notes from a long journey, one that would take its creator from early experiments on mice and dogs to bizarre surgeries on monkeys—and a daring attempt to relocate the still-living brain.

"He tried to transplant a head?" I ask. He didn't try, Michael corrects me. He succeeded. And no one has ever really told the tale.

At least, not until *now*.

What follows is perhaps the strangest story I have ever encountered. It's ample proof of the old adage that the most peculiar tales are often the truest, and that the most haunted and fertile story-ground lies inside the human mind, with all its curiosity, desire, daring, and dread.

# MR. HUMBLE AND DR. BUTCHER

# INTRODUCTION

## Meet The Resurrection Men

*T*he brain: *three pounds of gelatinous convolutions and a hundred billion nerves,* invisible in its machinations but responsible for all we think, all we do, and all we are. So long as we have our consciousness, then *we* are *we*. Violence, accident, and disease may carve away at our tender bodies, but most people still understand the *self* as housed in the mind—the repository of our memories, our hopes and dreams. But if you remove the brain from the body that houses it . . . well, that's another story. In fact, it's *this* story.

Open your wallet and pull out your driver's license. Many of us have a notation somewhere on the plastic indicating that we are organ donors, meaning in the event of our death, our organs may be harvested for the sake of saving another's life. After checking that box, most people probably never give the possibility another thought. We gladly accept—we *valorize*—the transplantation of organs, but less than a hundred years ago, the mere idea would have seemed the demented imagining of a sick mind. To take a beating heart from a body

I

harkened back to god sacrifices; to remove a liver from the dead to sustain the living would have been met with horror.

For centuries, institutions like the Catholic Church and common decency refused to allow even human dissection, resulting in bizarre and mangled ideas regarding the complex workings of the body. Early anatomists rendered the womb as a vase; the breasts they attached by tubes to the ovaries (assuming that somehow menstruation and breast milk were linked); and the brain, our most precious resource, they drew as a porridge of sludgy jelly. The spaces between organs—the ventricles, those hollows through which the blood could circulate—*these* mattered. The blood, in all of its seeming significance, carried the soul of humankind.

Then came the eighteenth century, with its resurrection men. Europe's cities reeked of refuse and open-air toilets; milkmaids trudged up streets with their buckets all the day long, soot and dirt and flies smirching the cream they ladled to passersby. Given the bad nutrition, bad air, bad water, and general foulness of a populace unconcerned with regular bathing, disease was rampant. The peasant patient often found his way into the grave only to be dug out again. With no refrigeration and no body-donation programs, enterprising doctors relied on the dirty work of men willing to cast aside funerary wreaths, wrestle the recently interred from the earth, and retreat before dawn with cadavers they'd provide to young anatomists—for a price, no questions asked. It sounds macabre, but how else would a medical student learn about the body beneath its wrapping of skin?

Now the true shapes and functions of the organs could be determined: the liver with its two lobes, the four-chambered heart . . . But in which of these many pieces of meat, theologians wondered, did the spirit of a man reside? Since the time of philosopher-scientists like René Descartes ("I think, therefore I am"), this sacred space had been thought increasingly to dwell in the *mind*. Through the ministrations of anatomists and their resurrection men, the *mind* became synonymous with the *brain*.

Then came the Cold War years of magical thinking, when John Glenn left the confines of the earth, the Anglo-French *Concorde* and the Russian Tupolev Tu-144 supersonic jets took to the skies, and a new breed of resurrection men was born. Behind the Soviet Union's Iron Curtain, wards of isolated organs lived apart from their bodies as subjects of little-known experiments. By the late 1950s, strange black-and-white footage had leaked to the West, revealing seeming monsters: a heart living outside the body, lungs expanding on their own, a surgically altered dog licking up milk from its two joined heads. In secret laboratories, Stalin's scientists plumbed the depths of life's mysteries. They were not looking for the human soul. As good secular Communists, they interested themselves only in *life*: how to maintain it, how to isolate it, how to create it. They were interested, too, in control of the mind. Cold War research considered the brain to be a sort of radio receiver, sending and receiving electromagnetic signals. How did it work? Why did it work? How much of it did you need to survive? And what happened when the brain "died" but the body lived on? What about when the roles were reversed and the body alone gave out? Lives could be spared the slow degradation of the cancer that ate away organs—or the weakening of muscular dystrophy, or the stiffening of Lou Gehrig's disease—if only the brain could itself be moved.

And so, out of the midcentury spirit of desperate scientific rivalry, came an impossible dream: not a head transplant (per se), but a full-body transplant—lungs, heart, kidneys, and all the wrappings. It sounds too much like *Frankenstein*. It sounds like the fever dream of B-movie scientists in frightful labs. But in the end, this isn't a Frankenstein story at all; it's a Jekyll-and-Hyde story of a doctor with two selves, two impulses, and even two names.

# MR. HUMBLE AND DR. BUTCHER

Robert J. White, staunch defender of ethics, a good Catholic, and friend to two popes, liked to refer to himself (rather ironically) as Humble Bob. Young and ambitious, a savant so talented that Harvard hand-plucked him for a transfer from his university in Minnesota, White was interested in what happens in the case of multiple organ failure. A witness to the first successful kidney transplant, conducted by his friend and mentor Joseph E. Murray, White wondered why you'd trans-plant kidneys and hearts piecemeal when you could do all the organs at once by transplanting the head. His detractors, including activists for the ethical treatment of animals, called him Dr. Butcher, and laid at his door the unnecessary suffering of countless creatures and the fearful ambition of a man who aimed at playing God. White defended science as a practice above reproach—but he also made appearances on television and in the pages of *GQ* magazine, carrying a medical bag emblazoned with the name "Dr. Frankenstein." He pioneered lifesav-ing techniques still used in hospitals today—from brain cooling for accident victims to practical surgeries rooted in reality—but he also consulted for the second *X-Files* movie and inspired the sci-fi horror film *The Brain That Wouldn't Die*. White helped to found Pope John Paul II's Committee on Bioethics, belonged to the Pontifical Academy of Sciences, and was nominated for a Nobel Prize—but he also cut off the head of a rhesus monkey so that he might sew it onto a new and alien body, a trial run for doing the same to a man.

The surgeries White pioneered might seem to commence under cover of darkness, but in taking up his scalpel, he entered an interna-tional contest every bit as determined as the space race, a Cold War competition between Russia and America to overcome mortality and to bestow life. The leap from dog to monkey to man would inaugurate a four-decade battle against the limits of science—and clash against new understandings of animal welfare, White's own chosen faith, and a public reluctant to support the harvesting of organs from brain-dead patients or the transplanting of the thing that makes us *us*.

There is always a longing for a future *almost* within our grasp. "How many things are we upon the brink of discovering," asks Mary Shelley's Victor Frankenstein, "if cowardice or carelessness did not restrain our inquiries." Do we dare disturb the universe with our tech? The answer is yes, we do. From the iron lung to today's ventilators, from the first kidney surgery to innovations in gene therapy, from White's brain-cooling techniques to innovations in implantable neural networks, our medical present has been driven by daring leaps of the medical past. We have come to see as science what was once science fiction—and yet transplantation still tickles the senses with a combination of desire and lingering dread. When the mother of a deceased child listens to the heart of her baby in the body of a transplant recipient, whose heart beats in her ear? And if we have ourselves received the heart, the lungs, or the liver of another, does it change who we are?

This book tells the incredible story of a Frankenstein-like pursuit—a man's quest to perform the world's first human head transplant—and how this bizarre race inaugurated technologies that continue to save lives today. But it also explores a mystery that still begs solving: If you make a brain to live outside a body, what becomes of the self? Or as White put it, "Can you transplant the human SOUL?"

Dr. White's work serves as an extraordinary bridge between Cold War Russia and the United States, between science and soul, between the ethics of experimentation and the hopeful impulse to preserve patients from inevitable bodily decline. His story opens a window into the past, a time of zealous nationalism, of secrets and danger and spies—but also one of increased care for the rights of the forgotten, whether patients in irreversible comas or monkeys in labs. It's a tale about our greatest fears, our greatest hopes, and an astonishing invention that today saves cardiac patients and those on dialysis from certain death. And best of all, it's about the long, strange journey from science fiction to science fact.

# Chapter I

# FOR WANT OF A KIDNEY

We didn't think we made history. We didn't even think of history. We
thought we were going to save a patient.

—Dr. Joseph E. Murray, transplant surgeon

*December 20, 1954, dawned to thick falling snow. By midafternoon, Dr. Joseph E.*
Murray, a surgeon at Harvard's Peter Bent Brigham Hospital in Boston, stood in his kitchen with an ingredient list for eggnog. A balding, pleasant-faced man, Murray and his wife, Bobbie, were preparing
for their annual Christmas party, seventy-five guests strong—but the
phone rang in the hall before he could crack the first egg. "It's the pathology people," Bobbie told him. They both knew what that meant.
Murray dropped his whisk and threw on his coat. He cranked the
engine of his car, swerved out of the drive and onto icy roads. The
Brigham Pathology Department had a cadaver for him.

It's not often that a surgeon springs into action for the sake of a
patient already expired. But Murray wasn't thinking of the corpse. He
thought instead of a young Coast Guard member named Richard Herrick, who that December lay in fits of toxicity-induced psychosis in
the final stages of renal failure. Murray did *not* want the cadaver for its
organs, a natural assumption in an age when Western medicine has

proven its ability to extend life through spare parts. But in 1954, there were no spare parts; no organ transplant had ever been performed successfully. At least, not yet.

As the Christmas party went on merrily without him, Murray would spend the evening taking apart a fresh cadaver, painstakingly isolating and then removing a kidney—then repeating the process in reverse and putting the organ *back in*. It made no difference to the departed patient, but in three days' time, these hours spent in surgery might mean life or death; this was practice. On December 23, Murray and a team of fellow medical mavericks would subject Richard Herrick's brother Ronald, a Korean War veteran, to a dangerous surgery: they planned to remove one of Ronald's healthy kidneys and give it to Richard. It was to be the first transplant surgery of its kind and would inspire a race to other firsts. If a kidney could be moved, alive, from one body to the next, why not a heart? Why not a lung? For Robert White, a young medical student in the shadow of Murray's operating theater, the surgery would spark a singular and ambitious idea about bodies and their *brains*.

The human body is a messy, shifting organization of constantly dying and regenerating cells. The parts *are* the whole, and the slightest disruption can introduce a cascade of cell death. Consider your lungs: they must provide your brain with oxygen, or the brain will die. Yet your brain is necessary for engaging respiration. No brain, no breathing; no breathing, no brain. This same interdependence is true right down to the cellular level. When we die, we die all over, and for most of human history, the failure of even a single organ was effectively a death sentence. It's not that medicine hadn't tried to save organs and extend life; it's that it had tried and failed.

By the late nineteenth century, the introduction of antiseptic to combat germs, cleaner means of treating wounds, and neater ways of sewing sutures meant that surgery could be practiced with reasonable safety. With dependable anesthetic and much lower chances of infection, the surgeon could cut more deeply into the body cavity than he would ever have dared before. He could, in other words, do more than merely cut visible tissue, remove obstructing tumors, or carve off a limb; a skilled surgeon could correct the body, set compound fractures, and, in severe cases, operate on the organs themselves, to extract a burst appendix or perform a mastectomy, for example. But despite these (albeit grim) successes, removing any organ damaged it beyond repair. You could take out one that ailed a patient, but you couldn't pluck out a healthy one to give to someone else. Organs are fed by expansive networks of delicate blood vessels, and what you cannot "revascularize" — suturing torn vessels together without leakage—you cannot preserve. Transplant science could never progress unless this hurdle could be overcome. And as with most early attempts, the first experiments in doing so were messy, macabre, and almost universally subject to failure.

Alexis Carrel, a French surgeon and Nobel laureate, performed most of his surgeries on animals, particularly dogs. Revascularization only became possible in 1894 thanks to Carrel's experiments with silk ligatures; the fibers were fine enough that, aided by sewing lessons from an embroiderer, Carrel could patch up blood vessels with stitches so small they could scarcely be seen with the naked eye.[1] To avoid puncturing the vessel, he folded its tiny ends like a shirt cuff, stitching end to end so the blood would only come in contact with the vessel walls.[2] Once he perfected the technique, he set his sights on transplanting a dog's kidney. He had long been interested in treating kidney disease; patients regularly died of renal failure, and to stall that end, Carrel proposed experimental surgery. After all, you could remove one kidney without damaging the other, and—since the bean-shaped organs produce urine as a by-product of filtering toxins from the body—you could easily tell if your transplant succeeded by measuring urine output.[3] The cutting *out* worked pretty well. The *putting back in* was a more complicated matter.

Through his work with the vascular system, Carrel understood that the secret to keeping a kidney alive had everything to do with blood supply. One of his first trials involved the removal of a dog's kidney, which he kept isolated and artificially infused with blood in his lab before putting it back into the dog. When he put the kidney back into the *same* dog, it usually began working again, and the dog and kidney lived on just fine. But when he tried putting the kidney into a *different* dog, death usually followed. Not only did the transplant fail, its failure killed the host as well, as infection from the dying organ spread. Curious about the processes involved in this decay, Carrel performed the first of a strange and macabre series of experiments, swapping the limbs of dogs. Now living and working in New York, he opened the thighs of two dogs, one white and the other black. Soon, they wore each other's limbs.[4] Carrel told a colleague that such work was far simpler than organ transplants, though to unite the femurs to the socket he had been forced to ram a nail through the marrow cavity. The surgery caught the public's imagination, and fanciful sketches appeared in the *Washington Post*, giving the impression that the dogs had run about sporting their new limbs. In fact, they were never even able to move the new limbs—their nerve tissue grew back much too slowly, and after ten days, the dogs' legs grew fetid and rotten. Both animals ultimately died of infection. More trials followed, and more failures, too, the reason for which would not be discovered until 1924. This time, the breakthrough belonged to one Emile Holman, a surgeon who worked for Brigham some twenty-five years before Joseph Murray.

Holman's interest was in skin transplants, which had already been used to some effect for fifty years. As industrialization increased faster than workers' rights, accidents were common and often severe. In 1878, a laborer named Samuel Root suffered vicious burns in an iron-molding factory when a stream of liquid metal ran across his foot; other unlucky workers became caught in machines and had clothes and skin ripped away.[5] With enough of the body's protecting layers of skin burned or missing, a patient would die—and many did. However, a few surgeons risked trying to cover wounds with additional skin in hopes that they would heal over. Historian Susan E. Lederer even recounts tales of superannuated nineteenth-century surgeries where skin from two hundred different people combined to rebuild a single woman's scalp, a quilt of humans with the stiches still showing.[6] But as with all other transplants of the time, skin grafts never took for long. They puckered, pulled away, and died. Sometimes they held on long enough for the patient to recover their own skin; usually, they did not, and pain and infection ensued.

Blood typing had gained credence throughout the 1920s and 1930s, and by the 1950s had been almost universally accepted. This still-developing science gave Holman an idea. The *allograft*, or transplant of healthy skin from one person to another, had never been successful—not for long, anyway. But in Holman's day, children, with their grasping fingers above hot stoves and stumbling toes near open fires, were frequent burn victims. Perhaps a parental match would be almost as good as using the child's own skin, he thought, and so harvested grafts from a burn patient's mother.[7] The thinking might have been sound, but those grafts failed, too. Worse still, each time he replaced the child's allograft, it failed *faster* than before. The "destroying agency," Holman realized, came from the body itself.[8] Soon after, James Barrett Brown, a St. Louis plastic surgeon, confirmed Holman's fears: the "agent" was, in fact, an *immune* response. Somehow, the host body recognized foreign tissue, perceived it as an invading threat, attacked, and rejected it. The body seemed to know where it began and where it ended, and would accept no alien flesh. This meant sure failure for anyone hoping to transplant skin (or anything else) from another's body, a notion that, by 1940, had come to be accepted as fact. By 1950, Leo Loeb, a high-profile and prolific New York biologist, declared transplant prospects "hopeless" and a complete "waste of time."[9] His pronouncement seemed to be the death knell of transplant science for those practicing in the United States. And yet, at Peter Bent Brigham Hospital, the study of transplant continued. The hospital's surgeon in chief, Francis Moore, still believed there must be a way forward—and he brought Joseph Murray on board as an enthusiastic kindred spirit. Harvard's leading medical men looked on in pity and derision at what they considered the misguided captains of the university's very own ship of fools.

Then thirty-two years old and fresh from his training in plastic surgery, the young Dr. Murray remained unflappable about the possibilities. "I have been accused of being a pathological optimist," he would write in his memoirs years later.[10] He called his work in transplant "surgery of the soul"—it gave his life a sense of purpose, and no fear of skeptical colleagues would do much to shake his confidence.[11] He repeated Carrel's dog experiments—all except for the leg swap—and even transplanted cadaver kidneys into sick patients by inserting them into the thigh, where the bulge would be less noticeable and closer to the vents for urine. The point of such an operation wasn't true transplantation; a thigh kidney could filter toxins, but Murray knew the organ would eventually fail. The hope was simply that an extra kidney might take the strain off the beleaguered pair belonging to the patient, even for a short while. In most cases, however, it bought the patient only weeks, or days. Murray believed there must be a way to make the transplants work longer, but with 100 percent rejection rates, no one dared a full human trial. At least, not until Richard Herrick turned up at Brigham's emergency ward.

Richard had been an active and healthy twenty-two-year-old serving a tour aboard a Coast Guard vessel traversing the Great Lakes. In the fall of 1953, however, he fell suddenly ill, suffering weakness and dizzy spells. The crew sent him ashore, but his condition held on like a bad flu. Then, in January 1954, he woke to swollen legs and ankles. At first the problem was intermittent, and would gradually diminish throughout the day. But as the months wore on, the swelling continued through into the evening, the hot, tight skin making it difficult for Richard to walk. The pain sent him to see doctors, who diagnosed an excess of protein in his urine. It was a worrying sign: his kidneys were struggling to properly filter waste. Soon Richard's energy began to drain away; his mouth tasted strange and metallic, and he suffered from constant nausea and vomiting. Then, his urine ceased to flow. Richard was in renal (kidney) failure.

Our kidneys filter 200 quarts of blood in a single day, separating out toxins like urea (a crystalline by-product of protein), as well as chloride, sodium, potassium, creatinine (waste from the normal breakdown of muscle), and excess fluid, which exit the body as urine—up to two quarts of it *a day*. You don't need both kidneys to function; this redundancy is present in our reproductive organs, too (two ovaries, two testes), a quirk of evolution that acts like an insurance policy against injury. Except strangely, kidneys almost always fail *together*; the second kidney cannot help us if the other one becomes diseased. And when kidneys fail, the buildup of waste products in the body can be lethal.[12] If catastrophic renal failure (the term for a complete loss of function in both kidneys) occurs, the patient becomes 100 percent dependent upon dialysis, the painful and difficult process of mechanically purifying the blood, for the rest of his or her life. The individual must go to a dialysis center as often as three times a week to have their blood diverted into an external machine to be filtered before being returned to the body. Even with dialysis, many patients, especially in those early days, still died after only a short time. As it goes in the old rhyme, for want of a nail, the kingdom was lost.*

In less than a year, Richard Herrick's own little kingdom was in terrible shape. He went from a healthy young man to an emaciated patient in the final stages of chronic nephritis, an inflammation of the kidneys that leads to renal failure—and death.[13] With skin the color of bronze, he'd begun experiencing seizures and the onset of psychosis; he was restrained to his bed after biting a nurse. Even dialysis wouldn't save him for long.

As Richard's condition grew worse, the doctors transferred him to the Public Health Service Hospital in Brighton, Massachusetts, to be closer to family.[14] His eldest brother, Van, told Richard's physician, David C. Miller, that he'd do anything to save him, even if it meant giving Richard one of his own kidneys. No, Miller began to assure him, it would only be rejected—except Miller stopped midsentence.[15] He stood silent for a moment as an idea clicked into place. They couldn't use Van's kidney, no, but they *could* use a kidney from Richard's other brother, Ronald; the two men were identical twins. With Richard's kidneys literally on life support, Miller gave the order to transfer him to Peter Bent Brigham Hospital. He also called ahead to mention that Richard, unlike most unlucky patients, had a suitable donor.

---

*For want of a nail the shoe was lost.*
*For want of a shoe the horse was lost.*
*For want of a horse the rider was lost.*
*For want of a rider the battle was lost.*
*For want of a battle the kingdom was lost.*
*And all for the want of a horseshoe nail.*

—Anonymous

"It was the perfect human setup for our laboratory model," Murray would say in later interviews.[16] But should a team of surgeons put one healthy man at risk to save the life of another, even if it were his brother? And what gave Murray the right to decide?

## THE DARING OPERATION

Murray wasn't the fool his Harvard colleagues sometimes thought him to be. He'd had his first great transplant success a decade earlier during World War II, operating on a twenty-two-year-old airman who'd been burned on over 70 percent of his body in a crash in the Pacific theater. When GIs pulled Charles Woods from the wreckage, his lips, eyelids, ears, and nose had been burned off. Woods didn't have enough of his own skin left to harvest for grafts; he needed donors who could be relieved of enormous swaths. With no other recourse, Murray, then at Valley Forge General Hospital in Pennsylvania, used skin from cadavers from the hospital morgue's donation program.

Murray and his colleagues knew that once the host (Charles's body) realized an invader (the cadaver skin) had come, it would create antibodies uniquely prepared to target that invader. By Murray's day, surgeons understood that this immune response was the result of proteins produced by blood plasma cells to attack bacteria and viruses. Unfortunately, evolution couldn't afford to be choosy, so the proteins killed anything else that appeared foreign, too.[17] Still, a graft had to be attempted; without the necessary covering of skin to keep microorganisms out of his internal tissues, Woods would die of sepsis, or massive infection. Murray needed to keep Charles alive long enough for his body to begin regrowing its own skin, but the prognosis seemed grim.

Murray would have to keep cutting off and resewing skin patches, and he knew from Holman's work that the successive patches would fail faster than the first ones. Except . . . they *didn't*. A month in, Murray noted that the first skin grafts were still hanging on, alive and relatively fresh. It seemed a miracle at first, but Murray soon recognized the underlying principle. His patient's immune system had been so badly compromised that it could not produce antibodies to attack the new tissue. Something was suppressing the immune response. And if immune responses could be naturally suppressed, then surely they could be artificially suppressed. "I began to wonder," Murray would later write, "whether it would ever be feasible to go beyond the skin" and embed a donor organ within the human body.[18]

The story of Charles Woods's remarkable recovery made news around the world, appearing in *Newsweek* and attracting the notice of a surgeon named Francis Moore. Moore had treated the victims of the infamous Cocoanut Grove nightclub fire in 1942 (still the deadliest fire in US history with a death toll of 492).[19] Working with so many burn victims piqued the surgeon's interest in transplant science. When Moore became surgeon in chief at Peter Bent Brigham Hospital in 1948, he immediately established an experimental kidney program—and he courted Murray to Boston to take on its leadership. Both men believed there could be a way forward for transplants, but both also knew they needed a successful surgery to convince the world of organ transplant's viability. And they had not yet found a means of artificially suppressing the immune system, even if they believed it was possible. In order to fight the risk of immune response indefinitely, their first surgery needed genetically identical twins. Thus, it wasn't only Richard Herrick's dire condition that brought him to Murray's notice in 1954; it was the hale and hearty twin, *Ronald*.

Within weeks of Herrick's arrival at Brigham, a rapid battery of test results landed on Murray's desk. He'd performed seventeen formal tests to determine true genetic similarity between the twins, but only one proved conclusive: Murray grafted a small patch of skin from Ronald's arm to Richard's, and it thrived. But the nail-biting continued. As Murray made his way to the hospital on the morning of December 23, his favorite program was interrupted by a news bulletin: "BRIGHAM DOCTORS PLAN DARING OPERATION."[20] It might have only been the greater Boston metropolitan area, but Murray felt like the world was watching. A mistake here could shut down the lab, dry up funds, and set the clock back a decade—maybe longer—for the field of transplant surgery. To lose Richard would be bad enough, but not surprising, given his condition. The thought of losing the healthy twin, Ronald, was far worse. This surgery, Murray thought, might even be the first in modern medical history in which a *healthy* man underwent an invasive operation for no personal benefit. Ronald's sacrifice would only benefit his twin.

We are never ready for the future. It comes to us at the speed of life, and we take risks and make change in the space of moments. Murray and his team of surgeons didn't know they would be making history; it was far more likely that they were about to fail spectacularly. Because today organ transplantation works—because we've seen it done, heard of its success, even met the recipients—it loses the terror and magic it once possessed. Genetics can tell us what strange journey brought us our unique DNA, and studies of the human microbiome can tell us about the myriad living organisms inside us, from bacteria to parasites. But transplantation means taking the alien and placing it within the familiar. It means undoing the work of nature, isolating the veins, stripping the flesh, denuding the organ from its housing—and then rebuilding what nature grew from scratch.

Experimental surgery always carries with it both "can" and "should": the philosophical question of whether a thing ought to be tried at all. Transplant isn't just about practical medicine; it involves questions about bodies and souls—the animating principle, however you define it. What is a meaningful life? Who decides its worth and value? Who decides when it ends? In stripping away the boundaries of the impossible, Murray opened the door to something far more exciting—and far stranger—than he could have imagined. Transplant surgery asks hard questions about where the body ends and we begin. *Who* are we? *Where* are we? And what, for better or worse, does that mean for the future of bodies, brains, and the human soul? These questions might not have troubled Murray, who was too busy preparing for the practicalities of the morning's surgery. But they already troubled a twenty-eight-year-old medical resident roaming the halls just outside Murray's operating room.

## ORPHAN IN AN ALIEN LAND

Robert White elbowed his way through the crowded halls of Peter Bent Brigham Hospital. He'd heard the news like everyone else, but the thrill he felt went beyond novelty. He was older, and quite a bit poorer, than his fellow residents swarming the halls of the hospital two days before Christmas, abuzz with excitement about the surgery Dr. Murray was to perform—the one that would change everything.

White, a charming ex–football player in black square-framed glasses, was a Midwestern boy, born in Duluth, Minnesota, in 1926—the eldest son of Robert White Sr., a US Army Reserve Officer in the coastal artillery. Blue collar, middle class, and deeply Catholic, the boy's enlarged family included his mother, Catherine, and brother, Jim; his widowed aunt, Helen and her two sons (White's cousins Pat and Bill), all under one roof. Aunt Helen had been a schoolteacher; after a car crash took her husband, she became a helpmate to her sister, and the children became a rowdy bunch of playmates. Semi-chaotic, a little cramped, but warm and hospitable, the family moved to Minneapolis when White was fifteen, where he enrolled at DeLaSalle, a Catholic high school. That's where he met Brother Charles, the school's biology teacher. Brother Charles's final exam required the dissection of a frog, specifically the extraction of the amphibian's tiny brain. Square and stocky, White had until that point expressed more interest in sports than science, and had certainly never demonstrated previous aptitude with a scalpel. As he and his classmates began carving, chunks of frog brain spattered desks in messy, skull-crunched dribbles. But when Brother Charles came to White's table, he could see the slick membranes glistening whole, unmarred. "White, you should be a brain surgeon," he said.[21] White would tell that story for the rest of his life.

For the first time, White turned his attention to life beyond graduation, beyond Minnesota, too. The summer of 1941 allowed him to try out the idea: *Doctor* White, *Surgeon* White. But the world beyond Minneapolis's Washburn Avenue was heading into chaos. Hitler had invaded Poland, and both France and Britain declared war on Germany. In September 1941, the start of White's sophomore year at DeLaSalle, American reserves were called to duty, and Robert White Sr. received his marching orders. Without yet declaring war, we were at war.

The Neutrality Acts of the 1930s prohibited the United States from supplying munitions to the Allies, but America had become a supply line, ferrying money, weapons, and vital goods to Europe.[22] Now Robert White Sr. would be one of over a million men in uniform headed in the other direction, on their way to the Pacific. His post awaited in the Philippines, where he was meant to take charge of coastal batteries in Manila Bay. It seemed a long, long way to go: another world, almost another planet, and White Sr.'s military pay would not wholly support the family. Aunt Helen managed to find work teaching elementary school, and White and his brother took after-school jobs on the railway. September slipped into October with only bad news on the reels. They lit candles in the chilly alcoves of the local parish church and prayed hostilities didn't escalate. Everyone awaited letters home.

*September 4, 1941:* "Woke this A.M. to see a U.S. destroyer traveling beside us . . ." White Sr. wrote in his diary. *September 5:* "Our cruiser stays with us, traveling first on one side and then the other. Most comforting though . . . Wish Helen knew how swell her thoughtful writing kit has been." By the sixth, water had been conserved and showers shut off. Storms arrived and the seas rolled, and reports began circulating that an American destroyer had been attacked in the Atlantic. That Saturday, White Sr. repeated a news story in his diary:

> *On the morning of September 4, 1941, destroyer USS Greer (DD145) enroute from Newfoundland to Iceland when she picked up sonar contact with a German sub . . . The destroyer made and held contact for 3½ hours when suddenly, a torpedo was spotted heading for the ship.*

Danger lurked everywhere. With 1,400 men on board, the vessel was a floating target in the midst of the Pacific, so it ran without lights to avoid enemy fire. In the darkness, storms battered on with 30-foot swells.

They arrived on September 17 at Fort Drum, a small island at the mouth of Manila Bay. Heavily fortified and known as "the concrete battleship," it offered little comfort, and no joy to the men and officers of the 59th Coast Artillery Regiment. Days grew longer but more empty, until December 8, when the Japanese bombed Pearl Harbor. Then the war began in earnest, and though no one yet knew it, the South Pacific would fall into enemy hands. "I feel like an orphan in a strange world," White Sr. wrote on Christmas Day from a Fort Drum tunnel, their only protection against bombs. The concrete hold, like a bunker—or a coffin—kept them safe until May 1942, when the Americans lost Fort Drum. No one knew what became of White Sr.

There is no news like *no news*. The family in Minnesota waited. And waited. At last, the little bound diary, Aunt Helen's "thoughtful gift," arrived back at Washburn Avenue, carried by a military chaplain who'd been evacuated along with several high-ranking officials two months before the fort's surrender. The last entry begins: "The various unpleasant things I set down here do not represent a downcast or disconsolate attitude . . . but merely is a description for the future when this diary may be most interesting." It ends with "But of course . . . ," breaking off mid-thought. The silence of that last line hung over the family like a shroud. White's father had been alive when he wrote those words. He might have been alive still, desperate and waiting for rescue. When White turned eighteen at the beginning of 1944, he enlisted. It nearly killed his mother, but he meant to find his dad.

White graduated that June as valedictorian of his class, and soon found himself scrubbed and clean-cut and waiting on orders. He sat straight-backed and alert in the recruiter's office while the officer read through his files. High academic performance—and an interest in science—extraordinary aptitude, a quick and flexible learner. Like most young men, he should have been destined for infantry; the Battle of the Bulge raged on, and American forces bore the heaviest casualties.[23] Photos depicted heavily muffled men tramping through endless white paths and trees laden with snow, frozen foxholes strewn with dead and dying. They needed warm bodies, but they needed medical men even more desperately. "Wait here," the recruiter said. They left him to stare at the walls for half an hour. It felt like eternity. When at last the door opened, the man gave him a new directive: he'd be sent to the medical corps.[24] White shipped out to Indiana to undergo a wickedly intensive training course in laboratory medicine, from blood testing to water testing to the complexities of field equipment and basic first aid. He would end up not in Belgium but in the Philippines, the same far-flung corner of the world where his father had disappeared two years before.

White arrived first on the island of Luzon. His primary responsibility—to treat American soldiers suffering from malaria—merged with the ever-evolving demands of war. He spent his time guarding supply depots and testing water samples for parasites. It meant he didn't see the front lines; it didn't mean he avoided war's trauma. Amid grueling work hours and dismal conditions in the heat and damp, he spent his spare moments stopping in at prisons (now under Allied control) and medical stations looking for signs of his father. For White, this was Providence: he must be here for a reason. But the rolls never turned up his father's name, and the troops advancing into previously occupied territory hadn't found his father, either. What they did find were mass graves.

When Japan surrendered in August 1945, White was moved from the Philippines to Kyoto, Japan, where he joined up with a Red Cross hospital. Just nineteen years old, White set up a clinical laboratory in ten days and began testing water quality. He shared space with surgeons and other physicians, medics, and techs. All the while, the sick and injured poured in, many with limbs destroyed. Plastic surgery pioneers worked to re-create faces, building off the catastrophes of shell explosions and direct hits. How much could a man lose and still be himself?

To find some peace, White would walk to the Shinto temples just beyond the city. Red-lacquered shrines rose from the peaks and valleys of the forest, offing worship in ways both foreign and familiar. How, White wondered, could he reconcile the horror of war with a culture that worships? He'd learned enough of the Japanese language to understand that the people here had been devastated as well, and he began to reflect on his faith. He loved medicine, but could he perhaps serve people better as a man of the cloth? Two paths suddenly seemed open for him: one led to the priesthood, the other to the surgeon's table. But with atom bombs annihilating Hiroshima and Nagasaki, concentration camps disgorging emaciated women and children, and servicemen suffering physical wounds and shell shock, he knew his first choice was best. He wanted to save those lives, to save all lives—if he could.

He hoped, too, that he might still save his father's. But after several months in Kyoto, a motorcycle courier arrived with a letter from Douglas MacArthur, a five-star America general and field marshal of the Philippine Army. The letter offered personal condolences: *We found your father's grave.* He'd lived only a few short months after the fall of Fort Drum, his captors leaving him at Old Bilibid Prison in July 1942. Within days of receiving the notice, White boarded a plane to Manila, stood at his father's grave marker, and wrote a short letter home: *I'm here with him.* Just a name on a stone with a number, and a mixture of pain and relief. Mission over, war over. He took the next flight home to Minnesota.

White's training in the military had offered him an education that far outweighed anything taught in a college classroom. He'd learned bacteriology, epidemiology (the control of diseases), bloodwork, and water testing—at one point after the nuclear strikes in Japan, he'd been asked to check radiation levels. He'd worked as a medic and a lab technician, and he'd performed field medicine, but he still couldn't attend medical school without a college degree. So White used the GI Bill to enroll at the College of St. Thomas in Saint Paul, Minnesota. In two years, he matriculated to the University of Minnesota to complete a degree in chemistry, and in the fall of 1951, White applied to the university's medical school.

The university boasted famous alumni and faculty, including Philip Hench, co-awarded the previous year's Nobel Prize in medicine for the development of the steroid hormone cortisone, and F. John Lewis, who would lead the first successful open-heart surgery in 1952. But success made demands. Many of the young cohort of eager students entering medical school with White weren't able to withstand the pressures of the program, and barely a year in, White found himself summoned to the dean's office. For a second time, he sat before a man perusing his accomplishments in silence. Were they kicking him out? "Robert, you don't belong here," the dean began, and White braced for bad news . . . "You belong at Harvard Medical." A full scholarship had been arranged for White to transfer to one of the best medical schools in the country—a shock of nearly overwhelming good fortune. White went on to graduate from Harvard with honors in 1953 and begin a residency in general surgery at Peter Bent Brigham Hospital under Francis Moore, literally steps away from the operating theater where a year or so later the first transplant was about to begin. He'd arrived exactly on time.

Boston, December 23, 1954: The Herrick twins' surgery began promptly at 8:15 a.m. For the first ninety minutes, Murray waited in an adjacent room, listening to a live wire transmission of the surgery on Ronald. His men needed to work fast, but without even the slightest room for error. One twin, one extra kidney: the doctors had only one shot. By 9:50 a.m., the doctors had isolated the blood vessels supplying the donor kidney, but they didn't dare cut them; Murray still needed to prepare Richard to receive the organ.[25] Unlike in early experiments, where the donor kidney wound up in a patient's thigh, this surgery required permanent implantation into the abdominal cavity.

Richard's condition had continued to deteriorate until even his mind was affected; Murray knew the toll of the surgery alone might kill him. Even putting him under anesthesia seemed a risk, but if they didn't act soon, he would die anyway. Once Richard was out and draped in gray-green sheets, Murray made the first incision into the flesh of Richard's abdomen. Once through the muscle wall, he carefully pulled back the peritoneal sac holding the intestines and appendix. In a series of carefully timed movements, he clamped the arteries supplying Richard's kidneys and leg with blood. Then, after a deep breath, he gave the word for Francis Moore to sever the blood supply to Ronald's healthy kidney and extract it.[26]

They call it *ischemic time*, the vital, adrenaline-soaked minutes between removing an organ and reestablishing blood to its tissues. Every muscle, nerve, and fiber vibrates like a trip wire; every motion must be choreographed; every beat and chime of the clock hands is watched. Moore delivered the kidney in an ordinary basin, wrapped in an ordinary wet towel; "humble transport for such precious cargo," Murray would later recall.[27] In that basin, clamped and staged, were the keys to Richard's kingdom. Murray placed the organ inside the abdominal wall, but could not establish blood flow until the surgeons attached the "native" vessels to the donor kidney. Next came the renal artery connection, laced into Richard's iliac artery. The clock struck 10:10 a.m., but still the clamps couldn't be removed. Thirty minutes ticked by, surgeons sweating under white lights and the pressure of public performance as radio stations for greater metropolitan Boston repeated the story over and over again, desperate for news.

Murray's team didn't complete the necessary connections until a quarter past eleven. "There was a collective hush in the operating room as we gently removed the clamps," he recalled.[28] Just the sound of machinery, the white noise of an operating room as blood flushed into the donor kidney. It swelled and turned pink; it had been without blood for an hour and twenty-two minutes, as had Richard's leg. All clamps removed, the kidney began to pulse—and to do its job. Within minutes, urine flowed so quickly through Richard's catheter that the staff had to mop it up from the floor.[29] The doctors implanted the free end of Richard's ureter into the bladder[30] and normal flow restored immediately. Murray breathed relief; they had made it over the first hurdles. Now they had to wait.

The Herrick twins would walk out of Peter Bent Brigham Hospital together only two weeks later, organ transplant surgery's first success. With the Herricks, two men developed from a single split egg, the kidney transplant meant meeting familiar with familiar. And yet when the vital fluids began to flow again, Richard still retained his two original kidneys in place. Richard now had three kidneys, his brother Ronald only one. He'd been awarded an addition rather than a replacement, and that carried with it inherent dangers. Murray worried the diseased kidneys would infect the new organ and wanted them out immediately. Dr. Merrill, Richard's more conservative original physician, felt they ought to remain. And so Richard's kidneys remained in his body like land mines, a death he carried with him for another year, when Merrill at last consented to their removal. Richard left the hospital after that surgery and continued to thrive; his psychosis had left him, and he returned to an active life. He married his recovery nurse and lived on his brother's kidney as if it were his own. "Man's Life Saved by Twin's Kidney" read the front page of the *New York Times*, followed by similar headlines across the nation (and beyond), each declaring the dawn of a new era. And oh, how it was.

Francis Moore continued to support innovation. He persuaded Peter Bent Brigham Hospital to develop one of the country's first intracardiac surgery teams, and today remains best known as Harvard Med's most inspiring teacher, perhaps ever in its history. He'd given Murray his start, a chance to prove himself, and under Moore's watchful scrutiny, Robert White Jr. became an able surgeon, too. Moore assigned White his first operation just months into White's first year of residency. It came as a surprise—he'd scrubbed in to assist with an appendectomy, and flirted with the attending nurse until Moore asked a more senior surgeon to stand down and give the kid a whirl. Alone at the table, with the nurse passing him instruments in rhythmic time, White came alive. Here, the raw nerve of being throbbed under his fingers. He'd never experienced that feeling before; he would chase that rush for the rest of his life. White performed the appendectomy, saved the patient, and stitched him up with perfect sutures. He would marry the nurse, Patricia, a year later. "I fell in love over the operating table," he would say—but White had also fallen in love *with* the operating table. It wasn't enough to perform surgeries. He wanted to invent new ones, to stretch the limits of what science could do.

But the question of "what science can do" ushers in a host of very complicated and even dreadful other questions—questions many surgeons weren't interested in pondering. By 1963, when the first international conference on kidney transplant took place in Washington, DC, a doctor stood up during a discussion of when to "harvest" an organ from a cadaver—that is, when is a donor sufficiently dead?[31] "I'm not going to just wait around for the medical examiner to declare the patient dead," he announced. "I'm just going to take the organ."[32] His sentiment wasn't new. Medicine had long been haunted by resurrection men who broke open recently buried coffins in the dead of night. That problem had been largely solved at the turn of the twentieth century through the creation of body donation programs, brought about in part by scandal (an affluent white politician accidentally ending up on the dissection table) but also by improved medical ethics and a new vision of scientific progress that encouraged public participation. And yet by going forward with this one surgery, Murray's team had inaugurated an era of "harvest men" and a need for new regulations, even new definitions of death itself.

To harvest life from the dead drives against some of our most carefully (if not always consciously) held beliefs. From the Christian believer in bodily resurrection who wants to "go to Jesus whole"* to those who fear bodies will be illicitly harvested and sold to the highest bidder, the transplant of tissue requires us to grapple with a most fundamental question: Where in this endlessly pulsating kingdom of cells and nerves does the living self reside? In health, our body and self may seem indivisible. But in illness, in death, don't we struggle against the weight dragging us under as if it is a thing separate from us? How, then, do we know *we* are *we*?

The disease that took Richard Herrick's kidneys would return to take his life eight years after his transplant surgery. In the months before his old kidneys were taken out, the infection had spread to the third; it had been killing the living man all the while. Murray went on to perform more surgeries, not upon twins but upon unmatched patients and donors as he experimented with ways of suppressing antibodies, from radiation to forms of chemotherapy. Eventually drugs would be introduced to do the job, and though by then Murray had moved away from organ transplant to the field of facial reconstruction, he would win the Nobel Prize in Medicine for his pioneering work.

White never developed an interest in kidneys. His passion had remained unchanged from the moment he lifted an amphibian's skull to

---

*Historian Susan Lederer asks, "What were the implications, for example, of transplanting tissues and organs if you believed that, on the day of divine judgment, you would experience the physical resurrection of the body? Whose body would be resurrected?" Susan E. Lederer, *Flesh and Blood: Organ Transplantation and Blood Transfusion in Twentieth-Century America* (New York: Oxford University Press, 2008), 186.

expose the tissue beneath. He left Peter Bent Brigham in 1955 to enroll in a neuroscience PhD program back at the University of Minnesota, and to become a research associate in the Department of Physiology at the Mayo Clinic—the near equivalent of two full-time jobs. As a surgeon, it meant encountering trauma all over again, not from weapons of war but from attempted suicides, car accidents, and other tragedies. The brain, like the kidneys, must have blood and oxygen to survive. He could stop the hemorrhage, could do his best to repair damage, but every second hacked away living cells of brain tissue. Some patients died. Others lived, bodily, but in a vegetative state. Exactly how much of this precious material could you lose? he wondered. Or, to return to the grim questions he'd faced during wartime, how much can you do without before you are no longer *you*?

White lost his first patient while at the Mayo Clinic. He would lose many more. Intracranial hematoma, the pooling of blood in the brain from ruptured vessels, claimed the lives of car accident victims. Cancers ate away at healthy brains and left their owners paralyzed or speechless after surgery. He'd been at patients' bedsides when the brain waves quit spiking, even though the lungs still breathed and the heart still beat. And ever so slowly an idea, informed by White's sense of duty, his own private grief, and his Catholic beliefs, began forming as he labored over his patients: "I don't think the soul is in your arm, in your heart, or in your kidneys," he would later write, almost as if he intended to marry medicine and the priesthood. "I believe the brain tissue is the physical repository for the soul."[33] If he could preserve that bulb of gray matter, if he could keep it alive, then he could preserve what was most sacred.

*What if*, he asked himself, *Murray didn't go quite far enough?* What if the answer to saving lives didn't lie in the transplant of single organs, one at a time—but in replacing all of them at once? "Life is precious and fragile, and often must be fought for," Murray would say at the 2004 Transplant Games, where athletes with new organs competed like Olympians. Dr. White did not want to transplant kidneys and hearts and lungs, however; he wanted to move the "self" from its diseased body into a brand-new one. While still a PhD student, he had decided upon what would become a lifelong goal: he wanted to transplant the *brain*.

# TWO-HEADED DOGS AND THE SPACE RACE

*A grainy black-and-white film shuddered across television screens in the last* days of May 1958. A man in a long white lab coat gestures to a corner, where a figure waits, shadowy and indistinct. He leads the creature into the light of a courtyard, revealing a strange composite body: a large mastiff dog with a strange and cockeyed mini-body projecting from its back. The second head lolls to one side, tongue panting, legs hanging askew over the shoulders of its larger mate. Offered a saucer of milk, both heads drink for an applauding group of onlookers; close-cut camera angles reveal the bandages and stitches. Cerberus, named after the mythical three-headed hound of Hades, parades before the camera, a surgically remastered two-headed dog.

No one speaks in the footage; even if they had, most of the wider world wouldn't have been able to understand. The film, and the physiologist behind it, Vladimir Demikhov, emerged from behind the Iron Curtain, inexplicable, macabre, and without much context. And yet the flickering images sent a tremor through the surgical world. The footage reached as far as Cape Town, South Africa, where Christiaan Barnard (already working on the first human heart transplant) felt compelled to try to repeat Demikhov's experiments. (Barnard succeeded, but the dog died, and he had an effigy stuffed and paraded about campus.) News of the film also reached the surgeons at Boston's Peter Bent Brigham Hospital, though Joseph Murray wasn't convinced of its veracity. Might it not be a hoax? Some dozen years before, Russia had released another film, its first ever produced for Western audiences, called *Experiments in the Revival of Organisms*. The film presented medical centers with whole departments dedicated to isolated organs: hearts beating on their own, lungs breathing by use of a bellows, the head of a dog supposedly kept alive by machines. This motley circus belonged to Sergei Brukhonenko, a man both hailed for his groundbreaking research into blood transfusion and, later, reviled (outside Russia) as a surgical charlatan. His experiments had been half-real chimeras. While he had successfully isolated certain organs, many of his other claims served only as propaganda, suggesting that Russian science would lead to human immortality. That didn't keep his footage from sparking fears of reanimated bodies, of life artificially extended beyond the grave—and the Cerberus film wasn't as easily dismissed. In May 1958, Demikhov gave a public lecture in Leipzig, East Germany, and would return there to perform several heart transplant surgeries on dogs in the months to come.[1] That following year, he took part in the XVIII Congress of the International Society of Surgery in Munich. In his presentations and papers, Demikhov revealed that he had been performing these kinds of transplant operations for four years, the first having taken place in February 1954—before Murray ever transplanted a kidney, before the West knew it was possible to transplant anything more than skin. What *else*, Western medicine asked, might the Soviets have done?

Many Stalinist laboratories operated quietly outside Moscow. The work remained shrouded in mystery, and unwarranted disclosure could mean imprisonment (or worse); scientists in the same lab limited conversation to the weather and the state of the roads, making progress on shared projects difficult and discouraging. That anything so gripping as film footage could escape from Russia unnoticed beggared belief. No—this was surely intentional. But what did it mean? The "leak" (if so it was) followed hard upon the famous words of Soviet premier Nikita Khrushchev, who in 1956 told Western ambassadors gathered at Moscow's Polish embassy, "Whether you like it or not, history is on our side . . . We will bury you!"[2] He meant to impress the assembly of the ultimate victory of socialism over capitalism.* Soviet supremacy, he insisted, was "the logic of historical development."[3] Demikhov's work sent the same kind of message, a warning to the West about the superiority of Soviet science. It shocked and dismayed, but it also begged for an answer. How would the United States meet such an unusual challenge? With only a spare few minutes of film, Cerberus and his surgical creator would inaugurate one of the strangest contests of the Cold War.

## WHAT IS SCIENCE IF NOT A WEAPON?

We have, all of us, grown up in a world of nuclear possibility. As late as the 1980s, students still performed air-raid drills, hiding beneath flimsy desks while pop icons like Sting released singles hoping "the Russians love their children too."† The military–industrial complex so

---

*Khrushchev later claimed he had meant "We will outlast you"; Americans, however, received the speech as a direct threat.
†Mister Khrushchev said, "We will bury you."
I don't subscribe to this point of view.
It'd be such an ignorant thing to do
If the Russians love their children too.

—From Sting's "Russians," 1985

completely anchors our understanding of the last century that it's only with difficulty that we imagine a world before it. Yet little of that extraordinary military apparatus existed before the *Enola Gay* dropped the first atomic bomb on Hiroshima on August 6, 1945. The publicly given reason for doing so was "to end the war," though firebombing campaigns had already ravaged Japanese cities, and Japan's hamstrung navy could no longer perform major maneuvers.[4] Historians continue to debate whether unleashing radioactive warfare had been a necessary step, but one thing remains certain: the atom bomb's sheer destructive force, mysteriously expanding from the telltale mushroom cloud at its epicenter, made it the most powerful weapon of psychological intimidation yet invented.[5] It sent a fearful message to the world about the United States' combined military might and technical superiority. That was, after all, the point.

Los Alamos Laboratory director Robert Oppenheimer himself had warned President Harry Truman against using new and untried power on human populations, insisting that "Mankind would be far better off not to have a demonstration of the feasibility of such a weapon."[6] It was far too dangerous to lift the lid on Pandora's box when the science behind atomic weapons already existed in the public domain. Scientific research (in the West, at least) relied on transparency, on sharing data through papers and conferences and conversations. The Manhattan Project itself may have been closely guarded, but the mathematical and tactical work had been crowdsourced among institutions, meaning certain discussions and even specific equations could already be accessed through papers and presentations. Given enough detail, Oppenheimer knew any qualified scientist would be able to work out the full formula. To make matters worse, a Canadian spy ring had already been passing atomic secrets to the Soviets.[7] As a result, when Truman informed Stalin that the United States had a powerful new weapon, talk didn't mean much.

Truman didn't trust his so-called allies in Russia; relations had been strained all through the Second World War. And so, under the gun from agencies critical of the enormous cost of atomic research and under pressure to prove the country's technical superiority to the Soviets, Truman gave the all clear to unleash this new weapon.[8]

The awesome, annihilating power of the bomb did more than end a war: it changed the role of science, which, writes Cold War historian Audra J. Wolfe, became a tool not only of war but of foreign relations. Among the American public, a climate of optimism developed, built on the belief that science had won the war for us, fostering a relaxed attitude toward our enemies and competitors. The United States, after all, controlled the brain trust of scientists, as well as the raw materials (stockpiles of uranium). Some researchers and government officials held less rosy views about both our superiority and the safety of our exclusive control. The most conservative estimates suggested at least a five-year monopoly on atomic ability. They were wrong. Soviets began testing their own atom bomb in 1949, and the gap closed faster as time went on. When the United States tested a thermonuclear (hydrogen) bomb in 1954, obliterating Bikini Island and spreading radiation sickness to unsuspecting people over 80 miles from the test site, we kept our edge for less than twelve months.[9] It didn't seem possible, but the Soviets had caught up to American ingenuity.

How could a war-torn country, still deep in debt, produce results so quickly?* The question haunted US officials. Mark Popovskii, a Russian journalist forced to flee to the United States for his reports about the Soviet government, described military laboratories "springing

---

*Despite most other Allied countries having their debts to one another wiped clean in exchange for their service in the war, Russia was faced with repaying insurmountable sums, evidence that relations between the Soviets and the West had already significantly deteriorated by 1945.

out of the ground like mushrooms," while Higher Examination Boards turned out up to five thousand doctoral degrees per year.[10] This wasn't mere saber rattling. If the Russians could prove their superiority in science and technology, they could control the temperature of the Cold War. If *my* science wins, went the argument, then that means my ideology's won, too—and both sides believed only one system could prevail.[11]

Across America, surgeons' changing rooms, the medical equivalent of the water cooler, buzzed with rumors about Russian medicine. Both Robert White and Joseph Murray had witnessed firsthand how military science could influence and catalyze medical science, reallocating resources toward plastic surgery to heal wounds and the study of pathogens that might make troops sick. Ever since the war, Russia's military tech "had come so far so fast . . . we wondered if there was some spill over in medicine," White would later explain, remembering the wild speculation of those days. "Maybe behind the curtain there were research centers that had cured cancer or found ways to replace the blood with artificial solutions."[12] American doctors were afraid the Russians were winning.[13] And through the occasional films, publications, and propaganda speeches that reached the West, Russia certainly tried to give that impression.

After the war, experiments in medicine redoubled. The Soviet Institute for Brain Research at Leningrad State University researched telepathy, or "biological communication," and attempted training programs to boost military personnel's precognitive abilities.[14] Fearful rumors suggested the Russians had even mastered psychokinesis for guided missiles, and that they dabbled in the occult. It might seem remarkable—even ridiculous—but the United States took these paranormal possibilities seriously. American scientists couldn't afford to be skeptical; no one really knew for sure that the Soviets *hadn't* made such breakthroughs. After all, a few decades earlier, splitting the atom had seemed just as magical, mysterious, and practically impossible.

The postwar era operated on two guiding principles. On the one hand, incredible hope for scientific (even pseudoscientific) possibility; on the other, an increasing dread that the Soviets would get there first—the science fiction trope that the enemy would somehow beat the "good guys" through mastery of technology. And so, when the Demikhov footage appeared, it acted almost like the mushroom clouds off distant islands. Whatever else occurred behind the Iron Curtain, the Russians were making monsters.

## PERFORMING THE IMPOSSIBLE

Vladimir Petrovich Demikhov was born in 1916—making him almost the same age as Russia's new socialist political system.[15] The child of poor peasants from the western Voronezh region (bordering Ukraine), Vladimir lost his father in the five-year Russian Civil War.[16] And so his mother, Domnika, found herself raising Vladimir and his brother and sister alone.

The Voronezh, largely agricultural, had a strategic location, offering transport of produce and grain from the countryside to Russia's industrial centers. Under the new regime, however, Voronezh (along with many other towns striving to industrialize) also became a center for mechanical engineering. Soviet propaganda made heroes of the laborer, villainizing the "leisure" culture of the bourgeoisie. Children were expected to work, and by the time Demikhov was thirteen, he was learning pipe fitting and mechanics at an assigned vocational school. Mechanism, with its gears and cams, fed his curiosity for process. How did things tick, he wondered, and could you "lift the lid" on biological processes, too? Tenacious even in childhood, Demikhov took investigation to extremes. His mother once caught him poised over the family dog, kitchen knife in hand. She'd narrowly foiled an anatomy lesson.[17]

Demikhov's interests followed those of aging physiologist and Nobel laureate Ivan Petrovich Pavlov (of Pavlov's dogs), whose "Bequest of Pavlov to the Academic Youth of His Country" called for the Soviet Union's young men to pursue "endless variations of experiments as far as human ingenuity permits," his words suggesting that wonders awaited those brave enough to pursue them. Demikhov was listening.[18] By the age of eighteen, he'd left his job as a mechanic to attend Voronezh State University, where, still intent on discovering the mysteries of the beating heart, he spent his nights working in solitude. He wanted to be a physiologist, like Pavlov; a subdivision of biology, physiology concerns itself with how things work in the living system. Demikhov believed that mechanism and biology could work together, and that a mechanical "heart" of pumps and bellows could, if perfected, function as a replacement for the organ itself. Just as an engineer could replace an engine, Demikhov felt sure he could replace a heart.

Demikhov's notebooks from this period present unusual exploratory drawings. He designed a pair of diaphragms, butterflied together and looking at first glance like the windows of a church tower. Four cannulae (thin, hollow tubes) connected the two diaphragms to the veins and arteries leading in and out of a dog's heart. Operated by an external electric motor, the diaphragms replicated the pumping action of the two cardiac ventricles by circulating artificially oxygenated blood through the cannulae and into the aorta, the main artery supplying the body with blood. In his third year of university, Demikhov felt ready to try out his machine. He captured a stray dog near campus and anesthetized it, and this time no one prevented him from opening its chest. His notes from that day read: "18:15 h death caused by cardiac arrest."

In fact, he had not technically "killed" the dog—or at least, not yet. He had a few spare minutes before the stopped heart would lead to irreversibly losing his patient. Demikhov removed the native heart and used venous cannulae to connect his mechanical device to the dog's atria, aorta, and pulmonary artery.[19] Working at speed, he switched on the electric motor, and the diaphragms whirred to life. Pumping continuously, the artificial heart fed blood back to the dog's organs and brain; the dog's eyes fluttered open and its lungs gasped a breath. The dog had made it through, its chest now sutured shut save for where artery and vein connected to the external machine. The animal lived for five and a half hours, despite having no internal heart of its own.[20] Demikhov had, effectively, brought a creature from the brink of death back to life. He was only twenty-one years old.

Building on his early success, Demikhov entered the University of Moscow for a graduate degree in biology and physiology. He owned no formal suit of clothes for his required school portrait, so he asked the photographer to superimpose one, effectively drawing in a collar and tie.[21] Unsmiling, with fierce eyes and a deep widow's peak, Demikhov had no hobbies outside of his work and no ambition beyond his lab. In 1940, he performed the world's first intrathoracic heart transplant in an animal (placing the heart within the chest cavity) and even attempted coronary bypass surgery—all on canines, and almost a decade before Murray would attempt kidney surgery on the Herrick twins. But despite all Demikhov's ambitions, these experiments would be interrupted by forces well beyond his control.

At the outbreak of World War II, he was called up to serve as a pathologist. His home region, so close to the western edge of the nation, fell to the Nazis during the German summer offensive of 1942. By the end of the war, 27 million people had died, and more than 70,000 Russian villages had been obliterated.[22] To make matters worse, the Truman administration was requesting payment for "nonmilitary supplies" to the tune of $2.6 billion.[23] Demikhov returned to his experiments in a country hamstrung by debt, but determined to prove its resilience—and, soon, its dominance.

By the early 1950s, Demikhov had performed over three hundred surgeries on canines and could perform an anastomosis (connecting two blood vessels together surgically) in 55 seconds.[24] He was not, however, considered a surgeon, as he did not have an MD. And though he'd finished the coursework, interruptions from the war and his own falling out with university faculty meant he hadn't yet earned his PhD, either. Despite this, he kept experimenting with little to no auxiliary equipment, often on a shoestring budget provided by his work in physiology. He eventually found employment at the Moscow Institute of Surgery. Even so, Demikhov relied upon the financial support of his wife, Lia, whom he married just after the war, to make ends meet. Both Lia and their young daughter, Olga, testified to his long nights away and his tendency to bring work home, so to speak, in the form of bandaged dogs that shared their tiny two-room apartment. Demikhov's mind never stopped, constantly revolving on unanswered questions about the beating of hearts and the sighing of lungs, about the intricacy of the brain and what it meant to the bodily system. Serious, ambitious, reckless: He was willing to do the unimaginable. Yet neither Demikhov's maverick medical ideas nor footage of his two-headed dogs would have shaken American confidence in their superiority all on their own.

On October 4, 1957, a 184-pound Soviet satellite streaked across the night sky and into orbit. Sputnik I's launch sent shockwaves of disbelief and dread across the United States and most of Europe. The problem wasn't the satellite itself, nor even its successor, Sputnik II.

The terror of Soviet space technology lay with the rockets that launched those satellites: if a nation could send something into orbit above the earth, they could no doubt launch much more threatening objects at targets far closer to home.[25] President Dwight D. Eisenhower had just inherited a terrifying nuclear stalemate, and now his rival, Nikita Khrushchev—widely seen in the West as unreliable, and dangerous—had rocket power at his command.[26] Sputnik's chief designer* had proclaimed upon the satellite's launch that "the road to the stars is now open," but Khrushchev valued rocket science more as fodder for propaganda.[27] He wasn't alone.

Richard Reston, son of *New York Times* journalist James Reston, had been in Russia with his father that fateful October. When he returned to England, he found his fellow university students voicing their dismay at America's fall from grace. "They considered it a great national failure," he wrote. "We had been taught that America had all the answers and suddenly we didn't."[28] The United States, which had seemed untouchable during the Second World War, had lost both strength and status literally overnight. Even Lyndon Johnson, then the Senate majority leader, felt deep misgivings. "In the open West, you learn to live closely with the sky," he later wrote. "But now, somehow, in a new way, the sky seemed almost alien. I remember the profound shock of realizing that it might be possible for another nation to achieve technical superiority over this great country of ours."[29] The rose-colored light of the 1950s had dimmed.

The Soviets chose a radio frequency for Sputnik I so that the clicks that reported its trajectory back to Russia could be detected by your

---

*Khrushchev obscured the man's name so that he (and the Soviet Union) could marshal the credit, though it's largely accepted that the satellite was designed by Sergei Korolev, a then-fifty-one-year-old engineer, heavyset with dark-circled eyes, who dedicated his life to the cause.

average shortwave radio, the kind people kept on shelves in their garages. This meant that after news of the launch, everyday people could tune in to the heavens and hear the faint trace of a Soviet creation sliding across the night sky. Experts in the field understood that this initial satellite posed no real threat to international security—indeed, physicist James Van Allen of the American satellite program felt cheered by the news of its launch—but what Sputnik I lacked in capability, it made up in possibility.[30] Russia wasn't a world away; it was right overhead. Pentagon lieutenant general James Gavin, who of all people was probably least surprised by the news, still felt it like a hole in his gut. "I felt crushed," he recalled, while his colleague John Bruce Medaris exclaimed, "Those damn bastards!"[31] We had underestimated the Soviets. Now the scramble was on—not to beat the Russians, but to catch up. The space race had begun, and already, the United States was losing.

At first blush, Demikhov's dog heads and the launch of a Soviet satellite don't appear to have much in common. One has to do with medical science (however macabre and bizarre), the other with rockets and weaponry. And while Demikhov's Cerberus experiment had turned heads the world over, they were almost exclusively the heads of men in the medical/biological sphere. Alexander Vishnevsky, then director of the Moscow Institute of Surgery of the Soviet Academy of Medical Sciences, had taken Demikhov on as a physiologist, meaning he would perform studies on animal functions, the results of which might someday have application to medicine. Vishnevsky felt such work was laudable and necessary, but his protection and support could only go so far, and the surgical twinning of dogs' bodies was not always well received. How long Demikhov would be allowed to continue was anyone's guess. In the supercharged atmosphere post-Sputnik, however, breakthroughs in Soviet science could give power, garner favor, and potentially provide funds and protection. They just had to be made *public*.

In 1959, journalist Edmund Stevens of *Life* magazine received an unusual invitation: he and American photojournalist Howard Sochurek were welcomed to document a Demikhov surgery. Stevens, who lived in Russia, had won a Pulitzer in 1950 for a series of articles for the *Christian Science Monitor* about life under Stalin, titled "Russia Uncensored." Despite being an American by birth, Stevens sympathized with the country he'd called home since 1934.[32] He had married a Russian, Nina Bondarenko, and would never return to live in the United States again.[33] Appreciative of the Russian way of life, he wrote stories for *Look* magazine, *Time*, *Newsday*, the *Saturday Evening Post*, NBC radio, and London's *Sunday Times* and *Evening News*. The invitation to write a profile was not new, but that the invitation came from Vladimir Demikhov, with permission from the Moscow Institute? That was novel, indeed. How could he refuse?

Stevens described Demikhov as "vigorously decisive," a man in utter command. The morning of the surgery, he presented his assistants and surgical nurse in turn, but the journalists could not help being distracted by the "patients," one of whom was barking incessantly. Shavka, a "perky little mongrel," yipped excitedly, floppy ears and pointed nose actively twitching and alert.[34] Her normally shaggy hair had been shorn away about her middle; she was soon to lose her torso and lower extremities, including all capacity for digestion, respiration, and heartbeat. Already anesthetized, Brodyaga, or "Tramp," lay upon the table next to her. He'd lost his freedom to dogcatchers, and would now serve as Shavka's "recipient."[35] While the journalists marveled, Demikhov called over another dog. Named Palma, she had a series of serious scars upon her chest from an operation six days previous; Demikhov had given her a second heart and altered her lungs to accommodate it. She happily nuzzled him, wagging her tail. "You see, she bears me no ill will," he said, as if answering Stevens's unspoken misgivings.

Demikhov scrubbed up for surgery on Shavka and Brodyaga. "You know the saying," he remarked in Russian. "Two heads are better than one."[36] Shavka, who had continued to bark all the while, was at last put under a heavy narcotic.

To the world, this was Demikhov's second two-headed canine surgery. In fact, it marked his twenty-fourth—two dozen surgeries (on forty-eight dogs) in five years. Demikhov had streamlined the process, and considering its complexity, the pace might appropriately be considered breakneck. Demikhov began by opening the back and side of Brodyaga's throat to expose the aorta, the largest artery in the body, and spinal column. He then drilled holes in the vertebrae and threaded plastic string through each. Meanwhile, a nurse wrapped Shavka's head in a towel, leaving only the shaved area accessible. Demikhov's assistant made the first incision to roll back the skin, and then Demikhov, wielding the scalpel with easy expertise, exposed the small blood vessels and tied them off, before carving away the rest of Shavka's body. The last stage involved severing ties to the lungs and heart, but this could not be begun until those delicate vessels and arteries communicated with Brodyaga's circulatory system. The easiest means of attaching the two together was to place Shavka on top of Brodyaga, just at the back of his head, closer to the larger dog's critical cardiopulmonary organs. Demikhov stitched them together, a canine jigsaw, using the plastic strings to anchor Shavka's head and forepaws to Brodyaga's spine. The entire procedure took less than four hours.[37] His first, in 1954, had taken twelve.

Finished with the grisly work, Demikhov removed his gloves. The idea for a two-headed dog, he explained calmly, had come to him ten years earlier. Now working on dogs seemed almost passé. "I have news for you," he announced. "We are moving our entire project to a wing of the Sklifosovsky Institute," Moscow's largest emergency hospital.[38]

They had outgrown the "experimental" stage, he claimed, and it was time to move on to human transplants.

Stevens knew of the successful Herrick surgery in Boston five years before. By 1959, Joseph Murray was experimenting with sublethal doses of radiation to keep non-twin kidney transplants from being rejected by the recipient's immune system; he proved that it worked—but the radiation itself did lasting damage. In the UK, Peter Raper of Leeds had used cyclophosphamide (a chemotherapy compound) as an immunosuppressant, but the patient had lived for only eight months.[39] Did Demikhov truly plan to operate on people, even though science had yet to find a reliable way to make non-twin transplants work? Demikhov waved away his doubts. They planned to establish a tissue bank, he explained, containing everything from organs to arms and legs. "Moscow is a huge city where hundreds die daily," he added.[40] Why shouldn't the dead serve the living? Demikhov gave Stevens a rare smile, and revealed he had a test subject already, a woman of thirty-five who had lost a leg in a streetcar accident. He planned to provide her with a new one. "The main problem will be joining the nerves so that the woman can control her movements," he added. "But I am sure we can lick that too."[41]

While they spoke, Shavka's eyelids fluttered. She could not wag her tail or control any part of Brodyaga's body, but she lapped up milk thirstily—although as her esophagus had not been integrated, the liquid merely dripped from her throat through a single inserted tube. Brodyaga woke, too, head bowed under the unaccustomed weight of the smaller dog. He required aid to eat and drink, as Shavka's paws now hung over his eyes. Demikhov called the two dogs "lucky beasts," honorably giving themselves to the pursuit of science, and maintained that these experiments would one day save human lives. The dogs would perish only four days later. Their awkward joined body made sleeping difficult, what with Shavka slumped over to the side, and a sutured vein between them twisted fatally. Demikhov didn't think of this as a failure, however.[42] Far from it.

Back at Brigham, Joseph Murray, reading Stevens's piece in *Life*, scoffed; the tissues Demikhov planned to transplant could never function properly, he grumbled. The dogs, after all, would have eventually perished for the same reason Alexis Carrel's dogs had at the turn of the century: rejection of the foreign tissue. Murray was now working hard on antirejection drugs, though he wouldn't have much success until the following decade; Demikhov couldn't expect favorable results unless, Murray added derisively, "the Russians have made some breakthrough we don't know about."[43] But as with the launch of Sputnik I, no one could be certain they *hadn't*. And the United States didn't plan to lose that wager a second time.

Enormous streams of funding poured into research and development. Since Russia had put up the *first* satellite, the United States would launch a *better* one. Since Russia put a dog in space (Laika, on Sputnik II), the United States would launch a chimp (named Ham). Stevens's *Life* magazine special proved Demikhov's proficiency with head transplants, and in the same spirit of creative one-upmanship, the US National Institutes of Health (NIH) began funding experimental laboratories. What the Soviets could do with dogs, went the logic, we could do with primates. And what could be done with primates could be done with humans. The United States and USSR had embarked upon an *inner* space race.

## GETTING FROM DOG TO MONKEY

In 1959, Robert White was four years into his neurosurgical fellowship at the Mayo Clinic in Rochester, Minnesota. Out of the operating room, he worked as a research associate in the state university's Department of Physiology. Days were hard; nights were harder. White worked in two worlds: groundbreaking research and delicate surgery. When he had time for sleep, he drifted off envisioning strategies for removing tumors from the brain.[44] Friends back in Boston described White as playful, charming, and happy to join the exploits of well-monied friends in New York City, where they fraternized with Rockettes from Radio City Music Hall. But the Robert White who emerged now, in the long hours of study and the longer hours of surgery, had a fierceness and a focus that would become a hallmark of his operating personality. "I would replay videos of the [next] surgery in my mind," he later told associates. "They were drawn from my memory of the surgeries I had done before. It was almost an obsession."[45]

His commitment to Catholicism had deepened, his training as a scientist prompting no crisis of faith. Quite the contrary: He viewed the operating theater as a "sacred space," a place where his God-given talents met their God-directed end.[46] Hadn't he been chosen? Hadn't he agreed, in the shadow of those Shinto temples, to give his life to the saving of others? Hearts and kidneys could not compare to the intricate nervous system; with his scalpel inside a patient's brain, he acknowledged, "I was millimeters away from causing death."[47] It might be playing God, but it was also *for* God. And perhaps that explained his extraordinary behavior in the operating room. His colleagues in surgery described him as a "vision of calm," and deadly serious. He never broke stride—not even when one of the staff dropped a syringe, the needle piercing White's shoe and his foot inside. He paused only to say, "Try not to kill the chief surgeon," before carrying on with the operation, carefully cutting away a deadly tumor through a peephole in the skull. (He didn't even remove the syringe from his foot.)[48] Once he was standing at the scrub sink before surgery, all the day's other concerns melted away. What replaced them was something more profound—and more ambitious. It was a private *joy*, a sense of doing what he was made for. To be operating in, and experimenting on, the complexities of the brain gave him an elation he'd never before experienced.

By day, he operated in the trauma unit and as a research associate in the University of Minnesota physiology lab. There, he could continue work on canine experiments for his PhD—the writing of which often took place in dead of night. In between, he attempted to be a father. He and Patricia had begun their family shortly after their arrival in Rochester: Robert (the third) was born in July 1956, Chris in January 1958, and, as the summer of 1959 approached, Patricia was expecting baby number three; there was plenty to be done around the house. Surgery, research, family—White juggled a PhD, a full set of patients, and a boisterous homelife by sleeping only a few hours a night. The habit stayed with him. He and Demikhov had that, at least, in common.

Demikhov's debut in *Life* returned White to his first thrill at seeing the two-headed Cerberus. Here was a man after his own . . . brain. For three or four years now, he'd been wondering, "Was it possible to maintain and sustain the human in the form of its brain after its total body had been sacrificed?"[49] He'd suspected so after seeing that first grainy film; now, with journalistic clarity and photographic proof, there could be no doubt about Demikhov's two-headed dogs. Back home with Patricia, herself once a neurology nurse, he talked about the possibilities. *I know it can be done*, he thought. The race was on.

White's PhD research didn't set about adding second heads. Instead, he focused on hemispheres, or rather, removing one hemisphere of an animal's brain and studying the results. Occasional hemispherectomies, as the surgeries were called, had been performed on humans since 1928, usually in extraordinary cases of cancer and tumors, or to treat severe epilepsy.* The results were mixed: sometimes patients recovered entirely; other times unusual consequences followed—loss of words or partial paralysis being the most common. Even now, we don't have a clear idea why, though possible reasons point to variations in neural plasticity (the brain's ability to adapt) and the age of the patient (younger is always better). In some cases, the two hemispheres are merely severed instead of one being removed entirely, usually to stop epileptic seizures that don't respond to drug therapy. The recovery rates tend to be even better, with minimal discomfort . . . and yet on rare occasions, bizarre symptoms follow, including what's been dubbed "alien hand syndrome," wherein a hand or arm (usually the left) appears to act of its own volition . . . in some cases smacking or strangling its owner.[50] The brain, in other words, is strange and wondrous (and sometimes creepy), and we know so little about it. Just how much brain did you need, White wondered.

White's team anesthetized rabbits, and later dogs, in order to remove one hemisphere of the brain: sometimes the right, other times the left. In most cases, the animals revived with little trouble—mostly only rudimentary problems of mobility—and lived more or less normal lives with half a brain. The spark of life seemed to reside in the consciousness of the remaining hemisphere, still encased in the animal's skull. Yet the Mayo Clinic was also a trauma hospital, and White a brain surgeon. Over and over again, he witnessed young accident victims, their skulls crushed or pierced, slip into comas, never to awaken. If you could survive with half a brain, then what accounted for those devastating results?

---

*The first was performed by Dr. Walter Dandy at Johns Hopkins Hospital, for glioblastoma multiforme, an aggressive tumor of the glial brain cells.

White had held a child's brain in his hands. He had heard hopeful parents beg him for answers: When would their baby recover? White pursed his thin lips during those fraught interviews; he suspected *never*. But do you tell that to newly grieved mothers and fathers? Or do you wait and let time reveal it in the days and weeks to come? White sometimes prayed with his patients. He stopped at the nearest Catholic church after surgeries and prayed there, too. But he knew prayer wouldn't change the outcome for a patient with a damaged nervous system. And the paradox nagged at him: if hemispherectomy had shown a person could survive on only half a brain, then it seemed the great enemy to regaining consciousness after head trauma wasn't the injury itself, but something else, something that happened post-surgery. White suspected the culprit must be swelling inside the spinal tissues that shut off blood flow to the brain after trauma, but he didn't know how to stop its effects with any calculated certainty. The answer would come from unusual quarters—and once again, it would have everything to do with dogs.

For several years prior to White's arrival at the Mayo Clinic, researchers at the clinic had been working on the problem of brain isolation. They aimed to isolate (that is, to remove and keep alive) a dog's brain in hopes of creating what are called "models." An isolated organ allows researchers to understand metabolic rates (the rate at which the organ consumes energy), how blood circulates through it, and other factors, without having to distinguish between the organ and the body (which has its own circulation patterns and metabolism). A surgeon might, without information gleaned from isolation studies (and extrapolated to humans), mistake how much blood a certain organ needs to be stable, and there was no room for such errors in complex surgeries. When White arrived at the clinic in 1955, his new colleagues still hadn't managed a complete isolation, accidentally squashing, cutting, or damaging tissue each time they tried. White was already known for his surgical precision; his hemispherectomies were practically works of art.[51] He soon joined veterinarian and senior physiologist David E. Donald's lab. Together, they began experimenting with cold temperatures, what they called localized hypothermic cerebral perfusion. They planned to put injury on ice.

## INTO THE DEEP FREEZE

Scientists weren't the first to consider the power of cold. *The Jameson Satellite*, a sci-fi story written by Neil R. Jones in 1931, had its protagonist deliberately frozen after death in hopes that the future would hold the key to immortality.* Robert Ettinger, considered the "father of cryonics" (sometimes mistakenly referred to as cryogenics) for his book *The Prospect of Immortality*, claimed to have been inspired by *The Jameson Satellite*, and a number of willing hopefuls have been frozen through the years. Dr. James Bedford, a psychology professor at Berkeley, was first into the freezer; he left money for a steel capsule and liquid nitrogen in his will. Actor and producer Dick Clair (*The Mary Tyler Moore Show*, *The Bob Newhart Show*, *The Facts of Life*, and *Mama's Family*) was next; Clair had AIDS, and hoped to be revived one day when a cure had

---

*There are plenty more examples. A pulp story called "The Frozen Pirate" by Russell William Clark appeared in 1887, its titular character a thawed and living relic of days gone by, while in 1898 Louis Boussenard's *Dix mille ans dans un bloc de glace* (*Ten Thousand Years in a Block of Ice*) introduced readers to another chilly form of time travel. Jack London's 1899 short-story medical thriller "A Thousand Deaths" tells the story of an emotionless doctor who repeatedly kills and brings back to life his own son, and H. P. Lovecraft's 1926 short story "Cool Air" tells of a man defying bodily decay through refrigeration.

been found.[52] So far, however, none have been successfully resurrected from their icy tomb.*

The medical case for cold storage had more modest aims: not time travel through deep freeze, but a slowing down of the body's biological clock. When we get cold, we shiver to generate heat. But if the body loses heat too rapidly, the nervous system begins shutting down. Dizziness and disorientation occurs, the body stops shivering, and, in an effort to keep the organs going, all resources for maintaining heat shift to the core. Blood (and oxygen) circulation slows, we cease to generate heat at all, and the heart stops. Hypothermia kills. Many thousands have died of cold in various military campaigns throughout history: twenty thousand, by conservative estimate, with Hannibal crossing the Alps, and a considerable number of Napoleon's men in retreat from Moscow.[53] Robert Falcon Scott, on his doomed expedition to the Antarctic, described how the cold affected the brain, causing confusion and sluggishness.[54] To turn the cold from foe to friend would require White to reverse this natural process. In localized perfusion, the aim was to lower the temperature of the *brain* separate from, and without lowering the temperature of, the *body*.

White and his team opened the dog's chest to gain access to the vascular system feeding the brain and used ice-cold saline to shock the system; the portion of the vascular system feeding the body, they left warm. The dog's brain entered hypothermia, bringing it to "cessation"— that is, the absence of cranial circulation.[55] No blood means no oxygen, and no oxygen means brain cells die. That had been the trouble with so many brain injuries, White hypothesized. Irreparable damage did

---

*In 2018, frozen coral reef larvae were "brought back to life" at the Smithsonian Conservation Biology Institute. But to borrow from *Young Frankenstein*, a coral larva, with very few exceptions, is not a human being.

not always take place at the moment a spinal cord injury occurred; instead, it happened three to four hours later due to inflammation—the body's response to injury by sending fluid to the site. Inflamed tissue squeezed the area, pinching and shutting off the spinal corridor that carries blood to the brain. Thirty seconds without oxygenated blood, and you lose consciousness; one minute, and brain cells die; three minutes brings permanent brain damage; and after five, death is imminent.[56] But under hypothermia, conditions *changed*. Though the saline bath would stop the blood from circulating for several minutes, the dog recovered when brought out of the cooled state. White felt an internal thrill. Slowing the brain's metabolic processes reduced the brain's dependence on oxygen. Surgeons could gain valuable time during surgeries, and if they cooled the spinal cord immediately after injury, it would halt swelling and prevent damage to nerves and brain cells. "We've done it. We did it!"[57] White would exclaim when remembering that moment of discovery—for the first time, he saw practical outcomes for his own patients: children who might be saved from quadriplegia, complex surgeries that wouldn't result in brain damage. The next step, surely, was to isolate the entire brain.

For White, a whole new world of opportunity had opened. If he could develop an extracorporeal (external to the body) means of cooling and warming the brain, it would be almost as if the body and brain existed separately. What if he externalized the blood and oxygen to the brain artificially? Then he could achieve a brain that lived *outside* its body.[58] But this would not happen at the Mayo Clinic. Pleased with their results, Donald and White continued perfecting their perfusion experiments on primates. The clinic saw in these experiments a future where human spinal injuries could be treated, and that became more important than pursuing the isolation of the brain. The practical surgical application outweighed the research agenda, but White had never considered himself only or even principally a surgeon. He was a surgeon scientist. And he wanted more.

We tend to privilege bolts of inspiration, hunches, and happy accidents. Historian Steven Johnson lists any number of favorite metaphors, from "flashes" to "brainstorms," in *Where Good Ideas Come From*, his history of innovation.[59] Innovations don't fall upon us from nowhere, however. They emerge from dark recesses of thought where clouds of half-formed ideas wait to be born. The brain-cooling experiment protocols didn't appear to White in a flash; they evolved slowly, aided by work of his Mayo Clinic colleagues. Now, after that success, White wanted to do something that seemed truly impossible, though only because no one had done it yet. If you began with the conviction that it *could* be done, then it was only a matter of time before it would be. White had already been turning the problem in his head, seeing experiments in three dimensions. He meant to pull the brain from its protective housing and, unplumbed from the vessels and arteries, maintain it artificially for as long as possible.[60] Demikhov had achieved a partial solution to the brain isolation problem; he'd discovered that a dog's brain (and its head and front paws) could be kept alive on the "life support" of another, larger creature. But he hadn't done the delicate work of removing the brain entirely, preserving its vascular system and blood flow all the while. And more important, a dog could never be a reasonable substitute for a human; to do true modeling meant applying isolation work to primates.

"Dogs are easy," White would say. Friendly, easy to work with, easy to train, inexpensive—and in every other way quite unlike a human. Their simple brains could never be a true substitute for our own. He wanted monkeys, and monkeys are *hard*. The difficulty and expense of procuring and caring for primates limited the work done with them in

Russia, where the blight of the Second World War and troubled social policies had crippled the economy. That made primates all the more important for White's experiments. You didn't put a man on the moon by suffocating dogs in satellite rockets, and you didn't change the world of medicine by teaching old dogs new tricks. But it could not happen at the Mayo Clinic, and it would not happen without funding and support.

## A LAB OF ONE'S OWN

Already an exceptional surgeon, and well published from his work at the Mayo Clinic, White found himself courted by multiple institutions even before the completion of his PhD. Offers generally came in one of two forms: he could join the hospital as a premier brain surgeon or as a premier neuroscientist, but never both. White turned each overture down. What he wanted, what he increasingly and desperately *needed*, was a place that offered space, flexibility, and room to work as a surgeon-scientist, just as Murray had, and just as Demikhov surely was. Departmental barriers acted as hurdles to his active mind; how could he pour his energy in only one direction? Then, in 1961, a year before White was officially awarded his PhD, a slightly unusual interview request arrived from Cleveland, Ohio, via a man named Frank E. Nulsen.

Eight years earlier, Dr. Nulsen became the Harvey Huntington Brown, Jr. Professor of Neurosurgery at Western Reserve University Medical School and University Hospitals of Cleveland. The trouble was, the medical school had no department of neurosurgery; he had been hired to build one from scratch. By the early 1960s, Nulsen had created a comprehensive neurosurgical residency program that included training at Cleveland City Hospital (soon after renamed Cleveland Metropolitan General, "Metro" for short), but the hunt for exceptional teaching talent never ceased. As an urban trauma center,

Metro was very unlike the Mayo Clinic. People traveled great distances to be treated at the clinic. Metro's emergency room, by contrast, catered to car crash survivors, gunshot victims, and poverty-stricken locals who could go nowhere else.[61] Such a constant barrage of often hopeless cases wore at the surgeons in residence, and turnover could be high.

A position at Metro might not have seemed, at first glance, to compete with White's previous hospital roles, but Nulsen had big ideas. "First," he explained to White, "you'll create a neurosurgery department at Cleveland Metropolitan." That alone was a remarkable offer: White would shape an entire department at the hospital, just as Nulsen had built the Division of Neurosurgery at Western. White would also hold an assistant professorship at the medical school, teaching and doing research in addition to surgery. But Nulsen knew his man, and he'd saved the best for last. If White came to Cleveland, Nulsen would give him the chance to build a brain research laboratory. That would mean finding his own funding through grants (true of most research labs across the country) and starting with only the smallest of rooms and a skeleton staff. But it also meant freedom to pursue both surgery *and* scientific research. White agreed immediately. He told Patricia they were moving a year early, with Bobby, Chris, their first daughter, Patty, and a fourth child, Michael, who was still in diapers. White would finish his PhD remotely. "And," he promised, "we'll get a bigger house."

The BRL, as White's lab was called, opened for business in September 1961, in a single room on the fourth floor of a research building on Metro's main Cleveland campus, off West Twenty-Fifth. The lab's previous occupant, Dr. Byron Bloor, had pioneered research into cerebral blood flow (measuring how much blood circulated in and out of the brain) using rhesus macaque monkeys. Dr. Bloor, White was told, had left a few pieces of equipment behind upon his transfer to West Virginia University; that should get them started until grant money began to come in.[62] Then, as now, most money for research at any institution came from federal sources, and in the heady days of the space race, Nulsen felt confident White would have no trouble finding funds.

White intended to use his new dual position to put neurosurgical faculty and residents in close collaboration with neurophysiologists, biochemists, endocrinologists, and even experimental psychologists and engineers.[63] He needed this breadth of expertise. He would begin with brain isolation—something that would require machines and apparatus to be developed and built, a fusion of biology and tech—but he wouldn't stop there. He had whole new procedures in mind, even a whole new field of neuroscience. White proudly claimed that his new lab would "write the book on neurochemistry"—in his isolation experiments, White would reveal basic but previously unknown facets of brain chemistry and physiology, the "chemical facts" without which we could not treat diseases like Alzheimer's.[64] But White had not lost sight of that first intoxicating glimmer of transplant surgery, nor what it promised for the transplant of the brain. Nulsen wanted a man who would take risks; he may have gotten the riskiest. White couldn't wait to get to work.

Still, it wasn't easy to transplant a family a twelve-hour drive away, despite his eagerness. And was he ever eager. The Iron Curtain had closed tight again, but White knew Demikhov had the jump on him. Had the Russian warehouse of ready organs come to be? Had Demikhov (a physiologist only and not a medical surgeon) managed to transplant the leg? And if so, with what results? Of the Soviet medical endeavors, there came not a word.

The same could not be said of the Soviet space missions. Each new launch strained international relations. In 1960, Eisenhower had proposed a nonarmament treaty for outer space (based on one developed for Antarctic exploration). The USSR hadn't agreed to the terms, however, and the Soviets made no attempt to hide the military character of their program.[65] They didn't hide their successes, either, no matter how unusual. By the time John F. Kennedy took office in January 1961, Soviets had orbited a curious menagerie of animals, including two dogs, a rabbit, forty-two mice, two rats, and a number of fruit flies.[66] Kennedy inherited both NASA, the newly formed civilian space agency, and the extraordinary pressure to make good. Just so long as the missions remained unmanned, NASA advisors maintained. The only thing worse than being second in space, they cautioned, was being first to kill astronauts in the attempt.[67] But that same year, Soviet cosmonaut Yuri Gagarin made the first successful manned Earth orbit, and soon Kennedy had doubled NASA's budget and declared the now-famous moon shot.

The following week, Kennedy's failed Bay of Pigs Invasion ended in the deaths and imprisonment of CIA-trained Cuban exiles.[68] Fidel Castro signed an agreement with the USSR allowing the Soviets to place nuclear missiles on Cuban soil. For thirteen days in October 1962, anxious faces watched black-and-white broadcasts. At last, the USSR agreed to remove its missiles from Cuba if the United States removed its missiles from Turkey. Full disarmament had occurred by the end of the following month. The episode was a necessary lesson to the Kennedy administration. Success in the Cold War was about playing offense and claiming defense; it made more sense to court rather than to threaten. Historian Audra J. Wolfe puts it best: the United States doubled down on its plan to "win the Cold War through peace, prosperity, partnerships," and, most important, "propaganda."[69] It was a war of rhetoric, one that aimed to capture people's imaginations—and to instill fear where fear was due. Kennedy had realized what Demikhov's Soviet handlers already knew back in 1959 when they allowed *Life* magazine to bring his two-headed dog into the living rooms of families in the middle of America: that innovation and achievement in the surgical sciences could be made into chess pieces for the advancement of your own agenda. Both space races, inner and outer, could be used to serve the state.

The brain feels no pain, though it is responsible for sending pain signals through the entire body. The brain pumps no blood, but without its impulses, the organs ultimately fail. This inordinately complex *thing*, more powerful than any newfangled supercomputer, more flexible and durable than its delicacy would suggest, somehow drives everything else. But unlike the black-and-white movies that show Dr. Frankenstein and his ilk stealing a pickled cerebrum and inserting it fresh into the skull gap of the recently dead, real dealings with the living brain required careful negotiation. The BRL team had questions to answer. How could they measure cerebrospinal fluid, a clear liquid found in the brain and spinal column, and keep its pressure constant so no damage occurred? What tools might be necessary to expose the basilar arteries, vessels so delicate and minute that they branch more intricately than tangled hedges? How much oxygen, how much blood—and at what temperature—would be consistent with life? Could all these measures allow them to sustain a brain mechanically in an extracorporeal system?

White understood that Metro would be a far cry from the hallowed halls of Peter Bent Brigham, and that Western Reserve University Medical School, for all its resources, was definitely no Harvard Med. But White would have staff, and space—and, most important, *monkeys*. That single room in a nondescript research building would grow to cover the entire floor, and would become White's second home for the next decade of long days and late nights. White coffee mug and white coat, black pipe and dark brows: Dr. White would continue his preparations for the removal of the primate brain. This time, he promised, the United States would be first.

# Chapter 3

# WHAT DO DEAD BRAINS THINK?

*The weather was fine for September. Robert White crossed the street from his bus* stop to Cleveland Metropolitan General Hospital under leafy shade and a pleasant breeze. Cooled by Lake Erie, Cleveland didn't suffer the drastic swings of season the way Rochester, Minnesota, had; autumn offered crisp mornings and bright blue skies. White had spent the late summer moving his family to Shaker Heights—a suburban hilltop boasting deep green avenues. White's little corner of it must have seemed almost bucolic. As promised, the house was far larger than the one in Rochester, a ten-bedroom brick Georgian with dormer windows, nestled into a thicket of greenery. The meadowlike side yard would soon be on rotation as a makeshift baseball diamond, football field, and skating rink for the White children and as many neighbors as could join in. Another baby was on the way already. Patricia had long since given up her work as a neuro-nurse to serve as chief manager of household chaos. White called their new abode a twenty-four-hour hotel-and-restaurant; friends and neighbors would occasionally refer to it as a zoo. Not that the children were left entirely to their own devices. Shaker Heights had some of the best public schools around, which, White would admit, had played into his choice of Cleveland over competing cities. Of course, having his own research lab at Metro helped, too. This September morning, White got up before dawn, caffeinated, and dressed for his first day, bound for glory in the one-room lab of his predecessor, Byron Bloor.

Bloor, the previous chief of neurosurgery, was born in Moscow. Moscow, *Idaho*. A solitary neurosurgeon at a hospital without a proper neurosurgery department, Bloor's work focused on cerebral blood flow and oxygen consumption: How do blood and oxygen circulate to and from the brain, and what happens when something goes wrong? Most people are familiar with the arteries that lead toward the heart; they might even recognize medical terms like *myocardial infarction*, better known as a heart attack, which can occur when these arteries become blocked. But the heart isn't the only highly vascularized organ in the body that can suffer infarction—nor the most important one. Not when you consider that signals from the brain control the heart and the lungs, and everything else. If you can have a heart attack, you can have a brain attack, too. Bloor studied *cerebral* infarction: blocked arteries leading to necrosis of brain tissue. We can live on surprisingly small bits of the heart, or, using technology (like Demikhov's external pump) to power the flow of blood and oxygen, with no heart at all. We *cannot* live without a brain. Bloor complained that no one took the pathology of cerebral artery blockage seriously—most doctors failed to assess how cerebral blood flow functioned even in a healthy body.[1] But White was fascinated by that question.

Standing at the door to the lab, White took stock of its steel tables, white shelves, sterile walls. The material left behind consisted of devices for measuring cerebral fluid: thin-walled 18-gauge needles, pipettes, glass globes, and plastic catheters. The inheritance might not have seemed generous, but the elements of experimentation were all still there. If he planned to remove a brain without killing it, White would need to be certain about how much oxygen traveled to and from the brain, and at what pressure, so he could keep this constant; otherwise, he risked shock followed by brain death. The lab, though small, offered a place to begin.

White's vision for the Brain Research Lab would ultimately involve a sizable staff. To start, however, his team would be far more modest in size. Anesthesiologist Maurice Albin had worked with White at the Mayo Clinic.[2] With serious features and still dark though thinning hair, Albin looked younger than White—though at forty-two, he was in fact three years older. Academic and erudite, Albin served as a "straight man" to the more dynamic and charming White.[3] It meant everything, White knew well, to have someone upon whom he could thoroughly rely—someone he could trust. The two of them were soon joined by Javier Verdura Riva Palacio, a neurosurgical resident originally from Mexico, whose steady hands and steel nerves would be second only to White's own.

The three, aided by nurses, made up almost the entire team for the first year, but still accomplished significant work—not least of which was designing a method of continuously measuring cerebrospinal fluid pressure.[4] Those early months set the ground rules for everything they would go on to do: White's research would have practical applications in the real world of medicine. They not only developed a method of measuring spinal fluid, they also worked out a way to "collect" it in an implanted plastic module—a technique that was soon applied to humans in clinical practice, useful for assessing pressure and diagnosing neurologic disorders.[5] Another soon-to-be useful technique came of White's work in creating visuals of cerebral circulation in monkeys, which he did by performing a brachial arteriography, a method of radiography imaging a bit like a moving X-ray. It would be adopted for use in human infants when seeing into their tiny systems proved necessary for medical intervention.[6] The team also performed surgeries to manipulate the brain stems of both monkeys and dogs, bringing them closer to their goal of isolating the brain. Meanwhile, White was simultaneously finishing his PhD, teaching neurology at Western Reserve University, operating on patients at Metro, and applying for research grants for his lab. He and his team needed money, they needed more space, and they needed staff. Their work deserved it, White made plain in his grant applications, because this wasn't mere philosophizing. He meant to *apply* his work, from dog to monkey to man.

White ultimately won a US Public Health Service grant in 1962 for the purpose of isolating the primate brain. He'd promised in his proposal that this research would allow him to answer a deceptively simple question: How does the brain metabolize energy? That is, how much energy (in the form of glucose) and how much oxygen does the brain need before being compromised? It was true, White's proposal argued, that brains had been studied before—but in situ, still inside the head, still attached to the body and its vascular system (even if parts of it had been tied off through ligature). "Unfortunately, in none of these biological models does the brain approach an isolated organ state," White wrote. To be really separate, and to really know how much energy the brain alone used, "all contiguous tissues competing with brain metabolism must be ablated," or cut away.[7]

Why was such information so important, especially to a public health grant committee? Because at this time, processes we now take for granted, such as how much of a drug might impact the brain or how stress might change us neurologically, were not well understood. Knowing how the brain dealt with external input (illness, stress, chemicals, pharmaceutical and recreational drugs) required a baseline; science needed to understand how the brain behaved without the interference of the body.[8]

Think first of your brain housed in its bony cradle, snug inside your head. Now think of it in isolation, unplugged from the information streaming in from nerves and fibers stretched to every finger and toe. The isolated brain served as a kind of surgical holy grail. White and his team wanted to know exactly what happened to those cells when they were smashed in a car accident or paralyzed by a stroke.[9] Why did the brain work? Why did it go wrong? What exactly happened when it died? Because no one had ever been able to look in on the brain's vital processes uninhibited and untethered from the body, its workings remained largely mysterious. The next steps would require creative imagination, but White had already laid the groundwork in his experiments with David Donald on spinal cord cooling. Just before White left Rochester, the pair had successfully perfused monkeys. Anesthetized with a 20-milligram solution of sodium pentobarbital, each macaque lay limp as they prepped it for surgery, shaving its neck and inserting a flexible tube into the trachea to provide oxygen. As happens in all instances of hypothermia, the monkey would stop breathing on its own if its body temperature dropped too low.[10] White made the first incision to expose not the spinal cord, but the carotid arteries, those great pulsing veins of the neck. Using a device called a cannula, which aided in connecting veins and arteries together, he pulsed blood from one artery into a small purpose-built heat exchanger. Ice-cold saline poured into the heat exchanger's flexible tubes, rapidly cooling the blood going to the monkey's brain but not that flowing into arteries downstream of the exchange. By cooling the brain, it needed less blood-borne oxygen to survive; by using the heat exchanger, the warmer body tissues were not in danger of hypothermic death of their own. White kept up the selective hypothermia for a full thirty minutes; of his eight subjects, five survived with no ill effects.[11]

Now in his own lab, White repeated the experiment with Verdura and Albin. It took them a full year of careful preparatory work, tweaking heat exchangers and assessing the resulting recovery outcomes, but they eventually perfected the technique. For thirty minutes, the brain might be thought of as functionally separate from the rest of its body. A secure supply of blood at a cooled temperature meant the brain could, with care, be excised from the body entirely. You could remove it alive, of this White was certain. He was about to get his first chance at performing breakthrough science—his first real challenge to Demikhov, he thought, in the inner space race. White was going to isolate the primate brain.

We call isolated hearts and lungs and kidneys "living tissue," but you can't make a heart beat without electrical stimulation, nor make lungs "breathe" without externally powered air pumps filling the sacs. Even Joseph Murray's kidney team understood that every second the organ spent outside a body, it was dying. For all the Russian surgeon-showman Sergei Brukhonenko's *Experiments in the Revival of Organisms*, dead tissue could not be truly reanimated, and the reason for this is more than mere mechanics. Each of our organs relies on something else to drive activity—to tell it to beat or breathe or contract. Each, in fact, requires a *brain*. Once you isolate the thinking, stimulating, processing origination of all this neural activity, however, a new question arises. White's work in the lab wasn't just asking "How will an isolated brain function?" but—more hauntingly—is this brain, on its own, a living thing?

To the naked eye, the brain appears as little more than a gelatinous soup. Science writer Sam Kean has compared it to a ripe avocado, scoopable with a spoon.[12] At its most basic, the brain is made up of a "lower brain" (with sections like the pons and medulla of the brain stem and the cerebellum), the "middle brain" (home to the thalamus, hypothalamus, pituitary gland, amygdala, and hippocampus), and the familiar and squishy-looking "lobes" (frontal, parietal, temporal, and occipital). The three parts are sometimes called the reptilian, mammalian, and primate brains. The lower brain controls basic body functions and movement; it's the part we share with various reptiles, from iguanas to Komodo dragons. The middle brain relays sensory stimulus and helps to capture and process memories and emotions.[13] But it's in the lobes, what we call the primate brain, where everything we associate with being human largely takes place. It's here where we get at the "self," that strange and amorphous thing that most people believe they have, and that frogs do not.* When we ask what it would mean to be a brain, alive but bodiless—or to wake in another body, or to be (like Jekyll and Hyde) of two minds and a single body—in every case, we begin with an assumption that the brain (or the mind) houses at least part of our personal identity—and, conversely, that it can be separated in some way from the body itself. Just months out of his PhD program, in his first one-room lab of his own, White was staking his reputation on his faith that this assumption was true. He operated on brains every day; every day, he had his hands on the pernicious boundary of mental and physical, mind and matter. That, after all, was his job.

---

*There are also, of course, people who feel that all animals have selves just as humans do. This is partly what motivates the animal rights organization PETA (People for the Ethical Treatment of Animals), and is a question that will take center stage in later chapters.

# A MIND APART

Just less than a year in Cleveland, and White's routine already bordered on predictable. He left the house before six a.m. every weekday and some Saturdays, making his way to a diner on Shaker Square. He'd taken not only to drinking coffee there, but also to serving it, stepping behind the counter to fill cups when the diner was busy. He knew most of the customers' names. They certainly knew his. He spent his days in operating rooms, and would come back on weekends to check on tender patients. He'd lost more than a few; Metro was a trauma hospital, and it bordered some of Cleveland's poorest and roughest neighborhoods. He'd seen plenty that was grisly, from gunshots to physical abuse. Yet he genially cajoled staff and teased students and nurses. He'd become well-known for practical jokes, too. A nonfatal car accident occurred one day near the butcher shop where White was picking up cows' brains for his students to practice on. He convinced his son Michael to dash one of the brains over to a late-arriving policeman, shouting, "Hurry, rush it to Metro hospital so they can put it back in!" White then called ahead to the emergency room to let them in on the joke. The officer arrived only to have the ER admissions clerk ask him, "Do you know which body this one goes in?"[14] White's levity may seem profoundly out of place, but he was also a pious, serious man. When he left work every day, he stopped at Our Lady of Peace for 5:30 Mass. "For my sins," he sometimes said, though the pilgrimage offered him much more. With its restive sanctuary, watched over by angels painted against a half dome of blue, the church became a place for laying the day's triumphs and tragedies before a higher power. Every day, White entered surgery to treat victims of trauma, or to excise tumors plunging deep into precarious cerebral folds. Every day, he was bound to lose someone. If the choice was between slightly disturbed humor and despair, then humor it would be. But he did at least try to set his own soul right before heading home to good-natured pandemonium.

White's older boys were six, four, and two; his daughter, Patty, had recently turned three; and newborn Danny had only just arrived. Keeping everyone fed and clothed was business enough. On Saturdays after Mass, White rounded up the four older children and "took over" the local supermarket—two full carts would become three and then four as the family grew. Patricia chided her husband (gently) about working for the city hospital; salaries were lower there, and it didn't help that White occasionally waived his fees. With so many mouths to feed and always more on the way, school clothes to buy, and general household upkeep and renovations, a surgeon's pay didn't go as far as it might. When White arrived home for dinner, often his only meal of the day, talk would turn to school clothes and supplies, the need for a maid if the household were to be kept from utter chaos, and the goings-on around Hough, a predominately African American neighborhood nearby. Patricia, a lifetime member of the NAACP, had helped to register voters there for the upcoming 1962 midterm elections, where many were supporters of Kennedy. Social justice mattered to White, too, who had been angling to bring more diversity to Metro. But no matter the topic of dinnertime conversation, some nights he couldn't keep his mind from wandering back to his experiments. He knew how to cool the brain—he understood, too, how to remove it. But keeping it fed by blood and oxygen after the fact would require more than surgical ingenuity. He needed a perfect machine.

After putting the children to bed, White retired to the study. He boasted sometimes that he read more than one book a day. It sounded like bluster to his colleagues, but his home office overflowed with print, awash in stacks of newspapers and magazines and little piles of books. Philosophy and research collided with fiction, including a dog-eared copy of *Frankenstein*. White remained in this sanctum from nine every evening until two or three in the morning, silent thought against a backdrop of whirring radiators (or box fans in the summer) and classical music. In the dark, he envisioned his work in three dimensions without referring to models on paper, suggesting that he possessed an eidetic memory, or the ability to innovate spatially. If so, it was a gift he shared with Leonardo da Vinci and Nikola Tesla. For White, this visualization allowed him to "see" surgeries, but also to see the kind of machinery a surgery might require. Though White had wondered about transplanting the human brain since his time at Peter Bent Brigham, the practical realities would remain out of reach unless he could accomplish these earlier steps. *What we need*, White thought, *is a sort of glorified lemonade circulator, the sort you see at gas stations.*[15] He might be able to keep a brain going indefinitely with something like that. But even as he took his turn getting up with the newborn, White knew that mechanical devices of that complexity would be difficult to build, hard to maintain, and prone to breaking down. What he needed was a different sort of machine; a machine that circulated blood without conscious prodding, that sent proper electrical signals about heating and cooling, that went about its business with almost no intervention at all. His infant son was just such a machine, all grasping fingers and toes, a perfect little wonder. White had always maintained that a body was just "a machine for the brain."[16] So why build something new when you could hook up a brain to another living *body*? That had been Demikhov's method, after all.

White caught a few hours' shut-eye before dawn, but was up and out when Patricia woke to attend to breakfast. He never needed much sleep anyway, especially when he had an idea to pursue. Back in his lab, White chose ten rhesus monkeys—five smaller ones between 6 and 8 pounds each, and five larger ones at 15 to 25 pounds.[17] He would take the brains out of the small monkeys and keep them alive by using their larger counterparts as a sort of life-support system, a primate blood bag. The "isolated" brain just needed a place to rest, where it could be bathed by circulating blood. The contraption White mocked up looked surprisingly crude, not so different from those heart and lung preparations from the Russian films. The naked brain rested on a suspended platform, still attached to a strip of skull bone, which housed electrodes. These were hooked up to an electroencephalogram (EEG) to check for electrical stimulation, evidence that the brain still lived. Under the little platform, White positioned a funnel secured to a reservoir (for blood) and a heating unit. The whole contraption resembled a glassless lava lamp with arterial tentacles for circulating blood from the donor body and back. After tweaking the model, the research team turned their attention back to the caged subjects of the experiment. The surgeons were ready.

January 17, 1963: White scrubbed for surgery. Together with Verdura and Albin, he'd previously cross-matched each pair of monkeys for blood compatibility. Now the smaller monkeys, soon to be mere brains, were given sodium pentobarbital and immobilized. They would not wake again in their bodies.

White and his team set about performing the perfusions on each pair, monitoring blood pressure and using oscillographic recorders to print and store data. Lee Wolin, an experimental psychologist, and Ron Yates, an engineer, had helped design the support systems, but in the operating room, White would rely principally on Verdura and Albin once again. Albin began by anesthetizing and shaving the monkeys, carefully removing hair from the entire head and neck. The blood-donor monkey would be shaved, too, in both groins, so the femoral artery could be more easily accessed. They carefully placed the first monkey's bald head into a fixation unit that resembled a three-toed claw. Its steel fingers secured the head at three points: a small wooden block sat against the roof of the mouth, and the double-pronged upper hinge of the claw fit into the orbital bone ridges, effectively inside the eye sockets. A joint on the contraption allowed White to rotate the monkey's head 180 degrees. To begin, the monkeys would be side by side, with the donor strapped into a specially made wooden "chair." The surgeons next inserted the femoral artery of the donor animal through a T-shaped cannula where it would be connected via tubes to the recipient. Both animals were then wrapped in thermal regulation blankets. White and his team needed to be sure the animals' temperature remained constant, as measured with an inserted rectal thermometer.[18] As the blood-donor monkey began to serve as a two-body circulation machine, White set aside his ever-present pipe. If his interest in the careful excising of tissue had begun in the Catholic school dissection room, then he'd been waiting for this moment for more than two decades.

Up till this point, the surgery had been simple: two monkeys, wrapped in blankets, sharing circulation through a tube. Now work could begin on the smaller monkey, where it lay upon its back on an adjustable miniature operating table. White made the first incision into the head. The cut extended along the angle of the jaw so the skin could be peeled back. One by one White and Verdura severed and removed the anterior neck muscles and those along the lateral surface of the neck bones. White severed the trachea next, and this, along with the esophagus, was lifted up and away from the muscles at the base of the skull.[19] Meanwhile, assistants continued to monitor the monkey's vitals. Blood pressure, temperature, oxygen levels: Everything, everywhere, seemed in good order. It was time to begin cutting away the face, the point at which the process, despite all its care and sterility, began to seem less like surgery and more like the work of the local butcher severing cows' brains for market.

White rotated the monkey onto its stomach to better reach its scalp. This was peeled away, along with the eyes, nasal tissue, and anything left of the facial structures. White opened holes in the skull and Verdura attached six stainless-steel electrodes to the exposed brain tissue with quick-setting dental cement. Lacking a tongue, mouth tissue, and scalp, the monkey was now a skull on a body, fed by the blood of its partner. They rotated the monkey onto its back again and stabilized the artery pressure. Then they removed the animal's lower jaw, ever careful of the cranial nerves; severing those could damage the brain. Several complex procedures routed the carotid arteries into another cannula, itself suspended from heavy wire overhead, so a tube could feed blood directly to the brain.[20] The process of externalizing blood flow had begun, along with preparation for an "extracorporeal" (outside the body) perfusion. Four more steps, and they would be through. White cut the spinal cord and separated the column between the C1 and C2 vertebrae, just at the base of the head. The body fell away. Then, checking that pressures in the cooled brain were stable, they removed the skull support structures. At last, suspended from a small strip of skull bone and housed in White's curious apparatus with its funnels and tubes, was a perfectly intact monkey brain. The operation had taken eight hours.

Images of the surgery reveal a bizarre, macabre, and yet strangely familiar sight. The brain's gelatinous mass doesn't hold much shape; a brain on a dissection table quickly flattens out. But suspended from White's apparatus, bathed in life-giving blood and cooled to avoid any damage, the monkey's brain appears in textbook perfection. The convolutions offer a beautiful topography, the vessels and veins standing out clearly—still pumping, still full of vital fluids. It doesn't look like gray matter at all, but flushed and pink. And more than this, the brain was still sending out electrical signals, just as any living brain inside any living body would do.

The signals blipped at intervals, appearing as peaks and valleys on the EEG printout like the scratching needles of a seismograph during an earthquake. By measuring fluids, White could tell that the brain was also consuming energy, "feeding" itself on glucose. Biochemical reactions to sustain cellular life were ongoing—the brain cells *lived*.[21] White scribbled furious notes. Albin and Verdura did the same. The donor monkey awoke and needed feeding; then the researchers watched and waited some more. Sheltered in White's apparatus, the naked brain percolated signals, manifesting as darts and dashes on graph paper; a blip here and there might be a fluke, an error of the machine itself. But the brain kept it up for twenty-two long hours. It was, without doubt, *ALIVE*.

White, heavily caffeinated and clenching his unlit pipe between his teeth, considered the output from the EEG. The different lobes had been measured independently—frontal first, then parietal, then occipital—both pre- and post-isolation. Whatever was going on inside the monkey's brain after it was severed from its body wasn't *the same* as what had been happening pre-surgery. The occipital lobe, responsible for visual stimulus, had bottomed out completely, perhaps not a surprise given that the brain has no eyes of its own. The parietal lobe showed a significant change in activity, too: where the pre-surgery graph indicated tight but mostly consistent rises and dips, the post-operative graph presented rising spikes and deep fissures. As this lobe accounts for sensory information from other parts of the body, this sudden divergence might suggest electrical activity with nowhere to go. But the frontal lobe, home to cognitive skills, memory, and problem solving, retained something of its original pattern. It had been a little forest of tight spikes on graph paper before the surgery; after, the spikes grew farther apart, rising and dipping languidly, but still recognizable. "We have demonstrated for the first time the survival of the isolated brain," White announced.[22] One of the neurophysiologists in the room concurred, even suggesting that the brain might be better off without its body. "I suspect that without his senses, he can think even more quickly," the man hypothesized. "What kind of thinking," he added, "I don't know."[23]

It was enough to write a first paper, which would appear in the prestigious journal *Science*. But it wasn't *enough*. Surgeries needed to be repeated to be perfected, their results replicated and confirmed. The isolated brain's activity began to flag, and so White and his team decannulated the donor monkey, reversing the brain cooling and suturing its wounds, effectively "killing" the smaller monkey's attached brain before it expired on its own. The larger donor monkey would be rested and fed to support another brain at another time. It was enough for one day, and the exhausted crew went home to well-deserved rest. It wasn't an end, however, but a beginning. Surgery began again, as soon as could be scheduled, on the additional paired monkeys, two by two as the weeks went by. Unfortunately, each of the remaining sets had to be terminated partway through surgery due to a perilous drop in the volume of red blood cells to the total volume of blood coursing through the semi-isolated brain.[24] White speculated that this was due mainly to not being able to properly stabilize the smaller monkeys as their temperatures fluctuated and they lost blood. He terminated each surgery before the donor monkeys (larger, more expensive, and more useful) could be endangered; all of the donors survived.

It may seem like a callous waste of monkeys, or at least of research funds, but in this, too, White's "inner-space" experiments kept pace with the *outer* space race. NASA had been sending rhesus macaques, creatures whose cognitive ability might be compared to that of an average toddler, on ill-fated test flights.[25] Of the twenty-five or so space program monkeys, nearly all perished in one way or another, like a NASA primate *Gashlycrumb Tinies**: some suffocated due to mechanical failure of life-support systems, one blew up during ascent, another burned on reentry, some were lost at sea, and several that did return died within hours from overheating and stress. You couldn't put human lives in danger, scientists and surgeons argued, but for any new development, there is a messy implementation period. So process was perfected with nonhuman primates.

Not that monkeys were the only ones dying for the sake of experimentation. Most of the early human organ transplant recipients—willing and desperate men like Richard Herrick—didn't live long, either. A rate of one successful isolated brain in five was, by comparison, excellent—but White had to do more before scaling up the experiments. The biggest threat to success occurred in the process of trying to switch from dual circulation (where the monkeys were connected but the recipient monkey still had a heartbeat) to singular circulation supported only by the donor monkey. So much cutting meant potential blood loss; White used a cautery tool to prevent excess bleeding, but the heat from the blade could interfere with the monkey's temperature. To help with the transition, White added additional features to the operation as the year waned, including two small propulsion units—one for arterial circulation, one for venous circulation—that could run independently from a 24-volt battery. He also had his engineer, Ron Yates, aid him in creating a purpose-built oxygenator for the

---

*"A is for Amy who fell down the stairs; B is for Basil assaulted by bears," and so on, through an alphabet of deadly childhood mistakes. Edward Gorey, *The Gashlycrumb Tinies* (New York: Simon & Schuster, 1963).

units to bubble air into the monkey's blood through a series of tubes. All together, these new additions provided a sort of backup circulation system in case the donor monkey began to fail. This way, the smaller monkey's brain would have continuous support, even as the surgeons worked to connect it to the donor. White's team could operate continuously for twenty-four hours. They were ready to try again.

White and his team would receive more monkeys for trial between 1963 and 1964. In this go-round, the donor now sat in a high wooden chair, the lab filling with white noise from pumps and motors used to bridge the gap from one body's circulation to the other. The new technologies extended the original lava-lamp contraption into a room-long geometry of million-dollar specialized devices, with a monkey at one end and a naked brain at the other. White had not quite built the automated lemonade circulator he'd originally envisioned. Instead, he'd constructed a laboratory cyborg: part monkey, part machine.

The resident doctors slept in shifts, one set of eyes constantly monitoring the experiments and attending to the strapped-in blood donor. The principal surgeons, White and Verdura, had been joined by fellow neurosurgeon George E. Locke, and Albin remained chief anesthetist. Together, they performed the surgery sixty-three times, and at last, success outweighed failure.[26] The introduction of artificial circulation kept the brains from degrading, and the EEGs demonstrated a marked leap in electrical impulses for up to twenty-two hours.[27] White and his team anatomized the brains following each surgery, staining them with hematoxylin and looking closely at the slides under magnification for the slightest degradation of tissue. The brain tissues appeared normal, even after hours of perfusion and isolation. At last, White had proof of electrical stimulation, proof of healthy tissue, and proof of repeatability. It was time to take the work of the Brain Research Lab public.

## DEAD BRAINS DON'T TELL TALES

By 1964, the United States boasted four neurological societies, but the Harvey Cushing Society was both the oldest and the most stringent in its membership requirements. Established in 1931 and with a prestigious and long-standing pedigree, the Cushing Society's annual meeting privileged communication of significant scientific developments.[28] This was, for a man like Robert White, the place to be heard. And so, on the twentieth of April, he packed his bags and flew to Los Angeles to deliver a shortened version of a paper soon to be published in the society's journal, complete with surprising (if somewhat blood-spattered) images of the successful brain isolation. The final image, displayed to the assembled audience via projector, offered the first proof of that coveted surgical grail: the isolated brain, denuded and separated from the body.

For the surgeons gathered round white-clad tables at the Ambassador Hotel, the first brain isolation offered a means of studying the brain's reactions to drugs, changes in temperature, bacterial infections, and more, without the diluting influence of an attached body. At last, they could probe the answers to questions like: What does the brain need metabolically besides sugar and oxygen? Are there chemicals produced by the brain itself, even without input from a body? What does the brain do to protect itself without its bodily armor?[29] They grew excited about White's perfusion technique, too; he wasn't the only one presenting on the use of cooling, but his tweaks to the mechanics presented immediate benefits worthy of emulation. There was just one catch.

"Everyone can think of millions of things to use it for," White explained, somewhat deflated, on his return to Cleveland. A million things, but not the one thing he'd performed the surgery to learn.

White's colleagues in the Harvey Cushing Society acknowledged that the blips on his graph paper pointed to electrical stimulus from the isolated brain. But they refused to call that consciousness. The EEG that so excited White was met with noncommittal shrugs. "Don't aim so high," they seemed to say. After all, the neurological community couldn't even agree on what constituted brain *death*; they were not prepared (or even very interested) in discussing which blips and bleeps constituted *life*.

Until the mid-twentieth century, brain injury led to a halt in respiration, as the damaged brain stopped sending electrical signals to the lungs. Death soon followed. With the advent of ventilators, which fill and compress the lungs on behalf of the patient, however, brain-traumatized patients could live on, aided by artificial machines. "Brain death" was first described as a concept in 1956, but even then, the criteria were sketchy at best. By the following decade, the newly available data of the EEG offered some help. An "isoelectric" signal—a flat line—meant no electrical information registered on the EEG; this became part of the criteria for brain death, along with fixed pupils, no reflexes, and no autonomous breathing. But that still didn't really answer the principal question: Is this person dead? Or only "equivalently dead," technically dead?[30] In a landmark French paper, neurologist Pierre Wertheimer of Lyon, along with two of his colleagues, decided to call the state of meeting these four conditions "beyond coma"—a prognosis of death, but not death precisely.[31] That seemed too far to go. A brain-dead patient might be "as good as dead," but that still did not make the brain-dead body a "corpse." On the flip side of the issue, White's disembodied brain might demonstrate EEG activity, one of the criteria for life, but none of the others: no pupil movement because no pupils, no breathing because no lungs—and in fact, no circulation without the help of the cyborg-like amalgamation of donor monkey and machine. White may have demonstrated miraculous things—the cooling of brain tissue to almost 50 degrees below normal without damage, for a start—but he could not prove that his brains lived, and the brains couldn't speak for themselves.

Or could they? Back home in his study, amid the scampering sound of many feet—the boys had recently discovered they could pick the pantry locks with a disassembled Bic pen to sneak midday treats—White sketched out a new experiment. He had a daring idea, but the process would need to be divided into three. First, he ordered experimental dogs, rather than monkeys, to be sent to the lab. Twelve in total, they would be paired just as the monkeys had been, as donors and recipients. Verdura and Henry Brown, a new neurosurgical addition to the team, may have wondered why the seeming retreat from primates, but Albin knew better than to question. Before it came time to experiment on his new canine patients, White returned to the Cleveland Metropolitan General Hospital surgery for stage two of his plan. It was time for a trial of his perfusion techniques where, and when, they mattered most.

When Frank Nulsen took a risk and hired White, it had been because he wanted a neuroscience department every bit as commanding as the one at Harvard. And perhaps for this reason, something unheard of transpired sometime between April and June 1964. A patient, whose case remains anonymized, came in for emergency surgery on a malignant brain tumor. While surgeons operated to remove the tumor, White's team cooled the patient's brain to 51.8 degrees Fahrenheit from its usual 98.6. At so low a temperature, White believed the brain to be in suspended animation, "like actors motionless on a stage."[32] The doctors halted the blood flow temporarily through ligature of arteries, allowing for better visual and tactile work—what surgeons called "dry field" conditions.[33] With blood flow resumed and the brain brought back to its warmer temperature, the patient woke with no ill effects.

The surgery made its debut a year later in the international journal *Surgical Neurology*. The first official clinical trial of perfusion on human subjects at Metro wouldn't be approved until 1968, however, and was terminated shortly thereafter for fear of lawsuits.[34] White's hypothermic experiments would eventually establish what remains the standard of care for trauma patients in the twenty-first century—but at the time, they were a novel curiosity.

On June 8, 1964, White gave his first-ever interview to the *New York Times*. He did so on the strength of and interest in the human perfusion he'd just achieved, but he spoke less about his recovering patient than about his monkeys . . . because the third stage of White's daring idea involved taking his work to the public press, where it could reach a larger audience.

"Though the benefits and hazards of severe cooling of the brain are a subject of disagreement among medical scientists," read the front-page article. "Dr. White is convinced it is one of the most potent tools yet placed in the hands of the neurosurgeon."[35] White described the "extraordinarily exacting and delicate surgery" required to isolate the monkey's brain, although he left out the more unpleasant details. The article went on to suggest that surgeons might someday keep a patient alive without either heart or lungs, preserving the brain through an independent circulation machine. It showed White, in other words, as a pioneer. Shortly after, White republished the isolated monkey brain experiment in *Nature*, a multidisciplinary journal with a far wider distribution that the Cushing Society's limited sphere. These first risky leaps into the public eye would set a precedent White would follow for the rest of his life: he meant to do big, groundbreaking things, and he would not do them in a quiet corner.

Back in the lab, his team was about to try something new—an experiment likewise destined for *Nature*. Come publication, the paper would bear the unlikely title "Transplantation of the Canine Brain."

White's monkey experiments had proven isolation was possible, but without a body attached, the brain's electrical functions had no real output and no ability to interact with the world. He intended, therefore, to abstract the brain from a small dog and implant it, vascularly, into a specially created pouch in a larger dog's neck. The recipient dog would look relatively normal, save for a bulge at the neckline. Meanwhile, the living second brain would function in a working body, a body that would be stimulated while White measured the brain's response through EEG. He had already solved the "no reflexes" problem. He'd discovered that ringing a bell close to the stump of a brain's auditory nerve initiated the same chemical reaction as would be seen in living animals—and now he had a means of long-term "storage," so to speak, in a living animal that didn't need to be strapped into a chair and chained to the tubes of an artificial circulation machine. Stranger still, after the first of the new transplants, the canine didn't reject the interloper brain tissue as it would a kidney or liver; the brain lived on, benign and still functioning, in the body of a German shepherd. The realization came as both shock and reinforcement; it might not be possible (yet) to replace the brain of one body with another, as Dr. Frankenstein had done (and the dog's second brain could not control its body), but should you manage to clear the remaining hurdles, the body would (in theory) accept its new master as if born to it. Art imitating life science imitating art.

White and his team sent their findings to *Nature* in 1965. Then they waited. And waited. White's publications in and out of academe, and his increasing media presence, meant the scientific community couldn't ignore him, but they didn't agree with him, either. "Oh that's terrific, the EEG looks great," he said, recalling his frustration in a later interview. "But do you know if that brain is thinking? Do you know if that brain is conscious?"[36] White said yes; his neuroscience colleagues said *not so fast*. It could be mere reflex, or some yet-to-be-explained electrical continuance. It could be anything. And their skepticism made him restless. While not quite antagonistic, the responses from other neuroscientists must have felt alienating. Summer had come, and White wandered about the yard in sweltering weather with his wife. Patricia understood the culture of medicine, and she was a tireless supporter of her husband's work. But eight and a half months pregnant with their seventh child, her back hurt and her patience was fraying. "How about a holiday?" she suggested. "Take the children with you."

So began a family tradition, not a vacation for White so much as one for Patricia; they called it her "privacy" holiday.[37] She stayed at home, and White piled six children into the family station wagon and set out for the Breakers Hotel, near the Cedar Point amusement park on Lake Erie's southern shore.[38] The resulting mayhem required unusually regimented solutions. White had T-shirts made with numbers on them and purchased a megaphone. Then he set the children loose for a week on the shoreline. He watched from under a beach umbrella, with periodic injunctions of "Number Two, you're too far out, come back toward shore!"[39]

Sitting alongside Lake Erie, White worked over the same old problem. Only 1,500 grams of weight and trillions of cells, the brain was responsible for both all he knew as a human being and all humanity understood of the universe.[40] He knew it was the seat of consciousness—he felt it. But while he'd been only too happy these past twelve months to push himself into the public eye, he'd been reluctant to say publicly all he had in mind. How do you tell the world that you dream nightly of severely damaged brains in healthy bodies, and severely damaged bodies with healthy brains?[41] How do you explain your interest, your obsession, with preserving life for those trapped souls? As White watched his children play, their active limbs in harmony with their active minds, it must have offered sharp contrast to the problem at hand. He needed to *prove* that consciousness could be transplanted, and the best evidence of consciousness was the sign of the body itself. Demikhov and the flash of grainy footage that, along with the Herrick kidney surgery, had whet his appetite for all science could do offered a possible solution. A year earlier, Los Angeles had seemed a long way to travel. But as he questioned how to convince his colleagues that the isolated brains lived on, he looked toward Moscow. Perhaps Demikhov, and his two-headed dogs, would have some answers.

In the stack of correspondence in his study back at home were some unusually formal letters. He'd put them off, given excuses. Now he considered them afresh. The letters came from the I. M. Sechenov First Moscow Institute, where some of Demikhov's experiments had allegedly taken place.

White had been invited behind the Iron Curtain.

# Chapter 4

# BRAINS BEHIND THE IRON CURTAIN
## (OR, SCIENCE, VODKA, AND PRETTY GIRLS)

*In May 1966, the Soviet Academy of Sciences invited a United States oceanography* research vessel to dock in Leningrad. The Americans hoped to join in the second International Oceanographic Congress, set to take place in Moscow at the end of the month.[1] The vessel, the *Silas Bent*, would carry the latest technology and thirty-four scientists—but before the crew could leave New York, the Soviet Foreign Ministry intervened. Their ruling: Should the *Silas Bent* approach Russian waters, it would be considered a military vessel, and treated as such. United States officials protested—the ship *was* naval, but equipped only with computers, no weapons, no guns—but to no avail. "She's the newest and best oceanographic ship in the world," claimed Washington's Naval Office, adding that the Kremlin was just afraid of seeing how advanced American technology had become.[2] The Kremlin saw things very differently. Soviet newspapers carried stories of espionage, with spies pretending to be scientists in order to infiltrate and steal secrets. The denial of the *Silas Bent* was seen as further evidence of the deterioration of relations between the United States and Russia, part of a steadily colder-trending Cold War, especially as the United States escalated actions in Vietnam, with 184,000 troops now on the ground and extensive bombing campaigns.

And yet in November of the same year, Dr. White flew first class all the way to Moscow with the blessing (and funding) of the Russian government.

Glasses clinked and jingled as, beneath the carpeted floor, the engines roared and whined in preparation for takeoff. Bright billboards might advertise the "extraordinary quiet" of newfangled jumbo jets, but the metal birds still rattled and banged their way skyward. White leaned back in a seat that looked like a club chair, in a cabin that looked like a cocktail lounge. High-heeled flight attendants who had passed the three-part test of being young, attractive, and single pushed carts laden with gourmet dinners on china plates and served champagne in crystal flutes. White's fellow passengers were dressed almost as glamorously as theatergoers. White had donned a good suit for the purpose, too, though it had to be let out a bit; he suffered from a yo-yo cycle of weight gain and loss as periods of intense work caused him to forget meals—and periods of downtime to remember *all* of them. He'd been putting on weight again, but at 60,000 feet and on his way to Communist Moscow, White didn't have much of an appetite.

The invitations began coming a year earlier, after his debuts in *Nature* and the *New York Times*. A Russian delegation visited White's Brain Research Lab, a rare occurrence but a welcome one at Metro. Afterward, they kindly invited him to come back with them. *Just being neighborly*, White assumed. Not so. Official letters followed. Perhaps the Soviets didn't want oceanographers, but they seemed very interested in the surgical and biological sciences. They had also invited Englishman Harold Hillman, based at the University of Surrey, someone with whom White would occasionally socialize at conferences, as their research overlapped. Hillman was a biological scientist specializing in execution and resuscitation (bringing back the near dead). "Death is not instantaneous," Hillman famously maintained. "It is a process."[3] A fan of Demikhov's work, and also of White's, Hillman was enthralled by the mystery science behind the Iron Curtain, full of barely comprehensible breakthroughs made possible by the juggernaut of government enthusiasm and relaxed ethics. But that hadn't been enough to whet White's curiosity. When the first letters had come in, he'd complained to Patricia, "Why would I want to go to this ugly country?"[4] In the end, White went because of Demikhov's work. He needed to prove that transplanted and isolated brains could think; he needed hard evidence. His colleagues at the Cushing Society would accept nothing less.

As a Catholic, White shuddered at the thought of Soviet antireligious sentiment. As a patriotic American, he felt real concern about finding himself in a Communist nation, especially one that thought of America as its chief enemy. It wasn't uncalled-for anxiety. A Harvard professor visiting Moscow a month before White's trip had been accused of espionage and forced from the country, and even as White was speeding across the sky, two American ex-servicemen were arrested while hiking on the Soviet-Finnish border.[5] New laws had been passed expanding what the Soviets considered "slanders" against the state, including "news spread from Western radio."[6] And perhaps most alarmingly for a traveling brain surgeon, Russian journalist Albert Laurinchukas was in the process of publishing a near 500-page harangue against the United States, accusing surgeons of performing dangerous experiments on Black and Indigenous American citizens.[7] The claims were mostly erroneous, but only *mostly*. After all, American history bore the taint of slavery as well as the systematic slaughter and displacement of Indigenous people, and the American present was a hotbed of racism and clashes over civil rights.* What would the Russians think of White, both a surgeon *and* a scientist?

And yet as another round of stewardesses appeared and disappeared, proffering drinks as the enormous airplane heaved across an endless ocean, White smiled and felt himself relax. Flying was his favorite mode of travel, after all, even with its bumps and bangs. Living in such style made you feel like another person, and played on his ticklish sense of humor.

"Long flight, eh?" a fellow passenger asked. "Business or pleasure?"

"Both," White replied with a sideways grin. "You see, I'm a funeral director."

He'd played that trick before. It drove Patricia crazy. Sometimes White posed as a country veterinarian, others as a writer, once as a rabbi. He'd fooled gentleman actor Robert Morley on a flight to a conference in West Germany—the Brit later wrote up the encounter for *Playboy* magazine. It had begun as a means of connecting with people, so his fellow travelers wouldn't be too intimidated to talk.[8] Along the way, however, it turned into something else: the freedom of hiding in plain sight, using his increasingly broad knowledge of everything to convince fellow flyers of his faked credentials. Or maybe he got the idea from the US officials who called on him before he left, men in plainclothes who suggested that he would be debriefed by the homeland when he returned, that he *would* give a full report of just what the Russians were up to. Either way, after a full twelve hours in the air, and more time spent changing planes on the ground, White landed at Moscow's international airport, a lone American abroad.

---

*Medical experiments had, in fact, been performed on the enslaved before the Civil War, and forced sterilization was secretly practiced on Puerto Rican, Black, and Indigenous American women into the 1970s. In 2020, reports of forced hysterectomies in US ICE detention camps demonstrate that these practices continue.

A delegation met White at the airport, a military base only recently turned toward commercial use. Some of the scientists could speak English, but an official-looking interpreter did most of the talking. White might have appreciated a moment to get his bearings, but none was allowed. His bags were collected for him and, with the interpreter explaining things on the way, he was rushed to a waiting car. "Stuffed in," he later recounted. It was as though they didn't want him to see anything they hadn't planned.

White peered out the windows as they sped down the highway past enormous concrete buildings—most with no defining features and all hung with heavy electric lines that cobwebbed between the structures. Cold. Bleak. Gray. "Which hotel?" White asked as they approached the city center. One of the welcome delegation smiled. Young. Blond. Attractive.* She may have been another stewardess. No hotel, she explained. They were taking White to the home of a scientist.

They arrived at a well-appointed home, and though it wasn't as big as White's house in Shaker Heights, the furnishings inside the place surprised him. There were paintings and musical instruments, busts and sculptures. What the exterior of Russian houses lacked in character, they apparently made up for in culture.[9] White relaxed, if only by degrees, and joined a large party for dinner.

White knew some of the attendees from their visit to Metro: they were scientists from the Institute of the Brain,[†] Moscow University, and First Moscow State Medical, what is today known as I. M. Sechenov First Moscow State Medical University ( or simply Sechenov). He would

---

*This would be a recurring theme in all of White's subsequent trips. He would be met, sometimes by civilians, sometimes by military persons, but always by beautiful young women. It has been suggested that after the first few experiences, White made sure to request it specifically: "It improved the view." (Interview, John Rinaldi.)
†Moscow Brain Research Institute.

meet Andrei P. Romodanov, a soon-to-be famous neurosurgeon, then a research academician who would serve as director of the Kiev Research Institute of Neurosurgery, organizing most neurological research in the Ukraine, for almost forty years. White himself would interview Romodanov for the Cushing Society years later, calling him one of the "most distinguished and outstanding neurosurgeon[s] in the world."[10]

White knew it was customary to drink with your host—vodka, obviously, given the circumstances—but he rarely touched alcohol. He toasted to be polite, and managed to get water instead for the rest of the meal. At least it *looked* the same. As the courses and cocktails continued, the interpreter remained at his elbow. White suspected the man was monitoring him, and that some at the table were government officials.[11] Still, he found himself most surprised not by who made an appearance, but by who did not. Vladimir Demikhov had not been part of either the welcome delegation or the dinner, and White wouldn't find him at the Institute of the Brain, either.

The next morning they traveled to the nearby institute by car in inclement weather and spits of snow. White suspected they wished to keep him from looking around for himself. The arrival was something of a surprise; he'd expected a research facility inside a university or hospital, but they disembarked in front of an enormous redbrick facade. White looked up at the arching windows and detailed masonry of a pre-revolutionary mansion. Like much of Moscow's center—from the Bolshoi Theatre around Red Square to Saint Basil's Cathedral and the rising domes of converted churches inside the Kremlin—the mansion had been preserved in its original state of grace. Built originally as a Lutheran hospital by a family of Russian-German merchants, the building had been seized when the Bolsheviks "redistributed" the wealth of the upper classes. By 1917, it had become the Institute for the Study of Occupational Diseases, but ten years later, the institute refocused upon the brain, especially the brain of Lenin. Its mission: To examine the anatomical origin of the "extraordinary genius of the leader of the world proletariat."*

The Institute of the Brain owed its genesis to neurologist Vladimir Bekhterev, but its establishment offers a cautionary tale about the troubled relations between Soviet science and politics. Bekhterev's work began early in the Cold War, when he implemented a lab for telepathy training; he remained an ardent believer in fringe science all his life. Such beliefs were surprisingly common at the time; deep suspicion of Western innovations and a political block on information coming into the country lent an almost Galapagos-like evolutionary quality to certain aspects of biological research. As part of his work, Bekhterev argued that outstanding people must have physically outstanding brains, and that you could "reveal the nature of genius and talent" by creating a pantheon of brains to study and dissect.[12] Unfortunately, he didn't temper his science to suit his patrons' politics. In an unguarded moment, Bekhterev diagnosed then-reigning Stalin as *paranoid* rather than outstanding. He soon died of "food poisoning," and German neuroscientist Oskar Vogt received the directorship of the institute and the honor of dissecting Lenin's brain.[13] Soviet science was political science, and that lesson was literally preserved in the very construction of the institute, where Bekhterev's own brain remained, dissected after his untimely demise. One must not tell inconvenient truths.

White was allowed to view much of the institute, though not the treasured Room 19, which housed Lenin's preserved brain. Instead, his handlers took him on a tour through the city to visit Moscow Medical Institute and a strange sideshow of labs. White later described seeing

*This information was helpfully provided by Maria Tutorskaya of the Russian Medical Museum.

dogs' heads lopped off and attached to devices meant to keep them alive. But reality didn't square with expectation. The dogs exhibited brain activity for only seconds after the beheading procedure, during which time they would respond to sound or touch. But then the brain simply died. White frowned; he had already done so much more in his own lab, keeping a brain alive and active for hours and days.[14] Were they hiding their best work from him? Though he never told White, Harold Hillman had been having similar misgivings about his own visits. "They were frightened to tell us what they did," Hillman complained. "They filled us up with vodka and pretty girls—they didn't actually tell us what they were doing."[15] By the time White left the institute, he'd begun to have a nagging suspicion. The Russians weren't interested in sharing knowledge; they were *seeking* it.

White hadn't seen anything particularly groundbreaking, but the scientists and surgeons he met at the different institutes were eager to know about White's lab: about his cooling procedures, and especially about his ability to keep a brain alive after the body had died. White didn't mind being forthcoming to a point; the state of the Soviet equipment meant they were well behind his work at home. But it raised questions. *Maybe the Russians want to live forever*, he thought.[16] Did they want a forever Lenin? A constant Stalin? Or was it something else?

White managed, at last, to lengthen his leash from his handlers, though he guessed government agents still followed him, dark-coated and familiar-looking men at cafés and around corners. He'd left his hotel and gone for a stroll in the cold to think and, more practically, to buy a hat for his balding head. But in his ramblings, the things he noticed most weren't what the Russians had, but what they didn't. Descending into a metro station, a visitor would see brilliant marbled halls, statues of workers seeming to hold up the ceilings, ornate finials, and beautiful tile work. The trains ran on time, the crowds didn't push and pull, and there didn't appear to be graffiti or pickpockets about. Here was a testament to beauty and culture and efficiency. But sanctions, debt, suppressed economies, and an isolation enforced from within as well as without had done great damage. The undeniable proof of transplanted consciousness that White hoped he'd find behind the Iron Curtain simply wasn't there; just stories sliced as thin as Lenin's hippocampus.

## THE TRUTH ABOUT SOVIET SCIENCE

Moscow in the 1960s spread out over some 750 square miles, lumbering and gray, its mood little cheerier than its architecture.[17] Elderly women would queue for hours to buy basic amenities from state shops, restaurants served unpalatable food due to rationing, and everywhere service was slow or indifferent.[18] It wasn't long before White realized the poor quality of everything he'd purchased there. The fur hat souvenirs fell to pieces, some before he got them home, and the same for the boots he'd bought for warding off the cold. Basic needs were hard to come by, even sanitary products for women; these were the conditions for everyday people in a country supposedly built on the Communist ideals of equality for all. Meanwhile, the Party, or its ruling elites, lived as if in a different world. British journalist Gloria Stewart reported for the *New Statesman* on private clubs serving excellent food and drink, with service that rivaled the Savoy in London, and "closed shops" that allowed Party members to buy Western goods like modern televisions that were denied to their fellow men.[19]

The medical establishment followed the same uneven distribution of have and have not. When White was afforded the opportunity to operate, usually to demonstrate a tricky neurosurgery technique new to his Russian colleagues, he did so in sterile and well-supplied operating rooms. The Communist Party privileged the worker: public nurseries took care of babies so women could (and would) work, and public health campaigns sought to eradicate disease through vaccines and control of vermin. Yet public hospitals were little more than gymnasiums full of cots for the ill and poor, with few medicines. They seemed to White like the hospitals of history, a reversion to pre-antiseptic Victorian days.[20] His concern that Russia would overtake the West evaporated further with every new scene. Researchers and doctors alike were just doing their best under painful conditions. The people he met were hardy and resilient, with a love of music and culture and literature. Whatever the government of any Cold War power might say, the Russians themselves were just people, just everyday folk. They weren't even irreligious; many of them were Orthodox Christians practicing in secret, and White managed to find his way to Mass. What he hadn't found—yet—was the man he'd come to see in the first place.

Back in the 1950s, when White and his Brigham colleagues viewed the Demikhov films, they had filled him with a mixture of fear and wonder. Those miraculous dog-head transplants had seemed to him, at the time, to steal the thunder of accomplishment from even Murray's kidney transplant. As with the space program, many had felt as though the Soviets were one step ahead, like a superior Bond villain somehow eluding the West. Demikhov's exclusive *Life* interview spoke of a confident scientific program—a safe haven for exploratory ideas. But Demikhov's reality was much more grim.

Scientists, as members of an educated class and so always under suspicion, never quite shook hands with the revolution. Though their deaths were later redacted from the public record, many thousands of researchers and academics were arrested and executed after 1917 as members of the Russian Democratic Socialist Party (later the Communist Party) made war against their own intelligentsia.[21] Physiologist Ivan Pavlov, the first Russian Nobel laureate, watched in horror. "If what the Bolsheviks are doing to Russia is an experiment," he would say, "it is one to which I would not even subject a frog."[22] Academies closed, starved of funds and also of food. I. A. Velyaminov, the founder of field surgery, compared his fellow scientists to doomed gladiators entering the ring: *Morituri te salutant!* Those who are about to die salute you.[23]

After Lenin's death, Stalin would make the metaphor even more apt. He expanded the gulag system: labor camps created by the Bolsheviks to serve as punishment for political dissidents, intellectuals, and the bourgeoisie. The gulag would soon hold scientists, philosophers, and academics of all stripes, as different factions sought to rid themselves of those who would not fall in line. It worked a treat. In the years 1937 and 1938 alone, more than 10 percent of the Russian population (in excess of twenty million people) found themselves carted away to camps where life expectancy equaled one winter.[24] By the end of the decade, most of the pre-revolution scientists were gone, having been killed or (for the lucky few) having managed to emigrate.[25] Those who remained were rounded up in locked-down labs and forced to work on government projects; if you did not produce the results demanded, you would be shot.[26] Sergei Korolev, who would later become the unacknowledged chief designer of Sputnik I, was arrested in 1939 and prohibited from seeing his family for five years.

And yet, the nation *needed* scientists. Russia couldn't compete with the West without them. Desperate to increase its output of researchers, the state opened universities and scientific institutes to peasant children despite their low literacy rates, few basic education skills, and oftentimes lack of common dialect. Old textbooks had to be thrown out; they were too complicated. New, simplified textbooks replaced them, and classes were shortened. Eventually, the state reduced school terms for graduate students, too, and these "half-baked" researchers, surgeons, and pharmacologists were "set loose" on an unsuspecting public, as journalist Mark Popovskii reported after fleeing to the West. In the postwar years, the number of Soviet scientists boomed to over a million. Meanwhile, Party comrades became heads of departments in fields they knew nothing about.

The Iron Curtain didn't hide Russia's scientific riches, but its poverty. The state worked tirelessly not to protect secrets from being stolen, but to convince the world that it had something to steal.[27] The wise researcher learned to misrepresent the truth of what science could do; if a higher-up wanted the impossible, from telekinesis to the revival of dead organisms, it was smarter to lie than to speak unwelcome truths. That meant failure was often imminent. Near the end of his life, a demoralized Pavlov wrote his letter to "the Academic Youth," urging them to keep pursuing science, even if, the subtext suggests, the state itself stands in your way.[28] Vladimir Demikhov would begin his most important book with this quote; he considered it a motto to live by—even if a man could die by it, too.

The serene and confident Demikhov who appeared in *Life* magazine as the darling of Soviet science was almost entirely fictive. Demikhov's family escaped the gulag principally by chance, but the genius that allowed him to rise from child mechanic to PhD candidate in physiology would also precipitate his fall. He was not a diplomat; he had little patience; he was not often well received by his colleagues. And potentially most deleterious to his career, he had a knack for disobeying orders. During the Second World War, Demikhov served as a pathologist and accidental expert on self-inflicted injury. Soldiers unable to face the horrors of the trenches would often shoot themselves in nonfatal ways; if proven, such an action would result in immediate execution. In his first defiance of Stalinist protocol, Demikhov refused to provide evidence against these men. He lied for their lives, feeling that his medical role should not make him an executioner.[29] This rigorous adherence to his own sense of ethics meant he failed to make many friends in high places.

Once the war ended, his meager salary came from low-level pathology and physiology posts he managed to land at various institutions. Demikhov's colleagues considered him fanatical, even dangerous. After his first trials transplanting the heads of dogs, Demikhov's problems started to come from even higher up. In the early 1950s, a review committee from the Soviet Ministry of Health labeled Demikhov's work "unethical" and demanded he cease operations. Alexander Vishnevsky, who had given Demikhov a post in the Moscow Institute of Surgery and considered him a friend, managed to ensure a stay of that order, but he was on borrowed time.[30] When Demikhov presented his work at the 1954 meeting of the Moscow Surgical Society, claiming that his small organ transplant laboratory was performing experiments on animals in the hopes of extending human life, no one took him seriously; the surgeons called him a quack.[31] Demikhov needed to prove his usefulness to the government, and he needed to do so quickly.

The most pressing question circulating among surgeons since the first appearance of the Cerberus films had not been *how*, but *why*? Why create a two-headed dog when there would never be a clinical application for the procedure? The answer was more simple, and more sinister, than anyone might guess. To be of use to Soviet interests, Demikhov figured he would need to gain an international spotlight with something sensational, something the government would see as useful in its propaganda contest against the West. Demikhov rightly suspected that a two-headed surgical enigma would provide all the same horror and delight as Sergei Brukhonenko's old *Experiments in the Revival of Organisms*.

When Demikhov bragged to *Life* magazine that the Soviet fatherland had a fully functional organ bank and a successful transplantation protocol that included limbs, he was, as in his military days, lying for his life. What he had was a small lab, and in it he was trying without much success to prove that suppressing the immune system for transplant wasn't necessary—even possibly a piece of Western propaganda. His real research had to do with hearts and lungs and kidneys, the same pieces of interior machinery that had fascinated him from childhood. He busied himself with the idea of grafting, a horticultural technique of joining two plants until they grow as one. Demikhov assumed that, with proper technique, a human limb could be forced to grow onto a new human the way a branch of one tree could be made to grow in another's root stock. The principle at work in plants involves tapping into the pith of a plant, where nutrients flow; in the human and animal body, Demikhov believed revascularization (the sharing of veins and arteries) would allow for the same.[32] But there would be no successful leg transplant and no magical ability to save limbs without immunosuppressants.* Russia may have been interested in tissue banks, but it had nothing like a fully operational unit. Demikhov had performed his two-headed dog experiments partly to develop his grafting ideas, but also largely as a publicity stunt. Its success can be measured by the fact that the footage was permitted to leave Russia and spread abroad. And for a time, it did stave off the Soviet authorities. It cost him in other ways, though.

Cerberus didn't just shock the West; it shocked people in Russia

---

*At the time, the Russians were mostly experimenting with regrafting hands and feet onto the same body from which they had been severed. When ischemic toxin (a substance that accumulates in tissues deprived of oxygen and which can cause fatal toxic shock) was discovered in 1972 in the labs of V. V. Kuzenov, Kuzenov himself would try to suppress the information as top secret.

as well. Demikhov's champion at the Moscow Institute was horrified and refused even to look upon the creature, and Demikhov lost his post within the year. He managed to gain a paying post at Sechenov, where a year later, on the prestige of the institution, he was granted permission to attend an international surgery conference in Munich. He went with strict orders: *Do not tell anyone of the two-headed dog.* Demikhov defied them and announced his findings at the conference, which published its proceedings in the West. It meant Demikhov and his strange surgeries now had credibility beyond Soviet borders, but also that he had violated his injunction to keep silent. Immediately branded "politically incorrect and dangerous," Demikhov should have faced arrest upon returning home for disclosing national secrets . . . but for once, he'd been right about the risk.[33] His work had created an international buzz, and soon *Life* magazine and the *New York Times* would be at his door. But even this success was remarkably short-lived.

The police did not come, but the Ministry of Health shut down his lab, and in 1960 he was forced to move to the Sklifosovsky Research Institute of Emergency Medicine in reduced circumstances.[34] By 1964, his groundbreaking revascularization work would be taken over by Vasilii Kolesov, who would win the USSR state prize in science and become famous for cardiovascular surgery in Demikhov's stead. Worse for Demikhov, his disruptive behavior stalled his application for his PhD, the one thing that could guarantee better pay and a more secure position. Broken, frustrated, and threatened with eviction from his apartment, Demikhov contemplated suicide. There are competing accounts about what stayed his hand, from the intervention of family and friends to the publication of his book on transplants and its translation into English and German to his induction into Sweden's Royal Society of Sciences at Uppsala. But belated recognition did little to salvage Demikhov's reputation in his home country. When White arrived in

1966, he expected to find Demikhov at an institute, a gifted researcher at the very center of Soviet science. He instead found an outcast.

The Khamovniki District lies just to the west of Moscow's heart, a section of town stretching along a bend of the Moskva River. After his first intense days in Moscow, White wandered its streets more or less freely (though still followed by less-than-inconspicuous handlers), marveling at how much history remained. Here and there amid the brutalist concrete structures, some housing research units of Moscow University faculty, were remarkable buildings that had survived bombing during World War II, bulldozing by Bolshevik reformers, and burning during the Napoleonic Wars. By odd chance, the neighborhood's churches had escaped the flames through their utility as stables for Napoleon's favored Arabian horses. Now they had found new purposes.

Just to the front of a hospital and ringed all around by an iron fence rose a cream-colored brick-and-mortar dome. Known as the Church of the Venerable Dimitri Prilutsky, it had been built in 1895 by Konstantin Bykovsky, a Moscow University architect, so that the poor could hold their loved ones' funerals close to the hospital in which they had died. Squat on its haunches with thick, simple walls, it still housed animals, but of a very different sort. Deemed "worthless" for use by the Ministry of Health, the building served as a laboratory for an all-but-forgotten Vladimir Demikhov.[35]

"I don't get many visitors," Demikhov explained, flashing a smile. More to the point, he didn't get famous brain surgeons coming from overseas. It must have given White pause: the man he'd come all this way to meet thought *White* was the celebrity. Here Demikhov was, waiting on his American guest with unbridled excitement as he escorted White around his experimental models—dogs with replacement organs—and described the work he continued to do even without institutional funds. Demikhov now made many of his surgical instruments by hand, and kept records in old board-bound notebooks with mottled black-and-white covers, the sort schoolboys carried.[36] And yet despite this almost complete lack of modern equipment, Demikhov had developed twenty-four different methods of providing a recipient dog with an accessory heart that he could nestle within its chest, twenty-two of which had succeeded.

White could scarcely understand. How could the Russian have done this, when his lab lacked a heart-lung oxygenator machine or the ability to carry out any cooling techniques?[37] White knew only too well the brain's demands for oxygen; to perform a heart transplant surgery without proper auxiliary circulation meant no blood would get to the head for a time. It should have resulted in mental deficiencies—that was the whole point of White's own incredibly complex machinery for isolation surgery. The longer an operation took, the more risk of damage. Demikhov merely shrugged. Without the tech, he'd done it by being *fast*. Possibly the fastest knife alive.

Demikhov had transplanted almost every organ he could think of, and he'd done it on a shoestring budget.[38] If Russia hadn't proven a treasure trove of secret medical riches, White knew it wasn't the fault of the country's researchers. Demikhov was an extraordinary talent, but one held back by political factions and by his own suspicion of Western medical advances into immune response. What *more* might the Russians have achieved if their scientists had been unafraid and well provided for? What had the starving of scientists stolen from the progress of the world? White had gone to Russia expecting a rival; instead, he'd met an eccentric whom he could almost call a friend. In the years to come, he would describe Demikhov as fascinating, gracious, and forthcoming in a world of secrecy. "The entire field should recognize him, but American scientists didn't know his name," White complained.[39] He'd simply been forgotten, the Cerberus surgery a quirk without practical application.

Demikhov told White that despite the slow crawl of Soviet medical progress, he *did* still entertain hope for a tissue bank. In fact, he'd started one for living organs like kidneys while at the Medical Institute. Perhaps he exaggerated its support and importance, but at the very least he was endeavoring to make it a reality.[40] He, like White, had one goal above all others: the preservation of human life.

White didn't speak to Demikhov about performing a human head transplant, though Harold Hillman would later winkle out White's impression: Demikhov dreamed of one, too.[41] In Moscow, in Kiev, in all the major cities with their major hospitals, lay brain-dead patients that Russian medicine could not save—only keep alive physically tethered to breathing machines.[42] *Here* were the real "banks" of human tissue. But for White, standing with Demikhov in the forgotten laboratory, there were more pressing concerns. Blame it on the Bolsheviks, blame it on the closed borders and close-kept secrets, but the results were the same: Russia didn't have the right tools, or even the appropriate textbooks, to treat patients.

"I admire the Russian people," White would tell anyone who would listen back in the States. He'd describe how willing ordinary citizens were to help a stranger, how prepared they were to go out of their way.[43] He'd struggled with the currency, and strangers had gladly sorted his change for the proper kopeks to pay the streetcar. From the warmth of his reception by Demikhov to his growing détente with his handlers, who seemed happy to let him experience the city on his own at last, White couldn't help feeling that the race between nations had been ill-conceived.[44] He wanted, more than anything, to see the free exchange of medical and scientific information. He wanted to *share* his research, not to hide it, wanted the inner space race against Russia to become a relay *with* them. Yet as White boarded the plane bound for home, he knew that both the military and the FBI awaited him, their only question: Were we *winning*?

White had set out for the Soviet Union to find a way forward for his work. But the trip had changed him more than he could have expected. For one thing, the inner space race against Russia was effectively over. White already stood on the precipice of greater (and better-funded) discoveries than his Soviet counterparts. The trip had not altered White's desires, but focused them—and meeting Demikhov opened up different possibilities. He'd been asking himself ad nauseam: "How can I prove that the brain when transferred or transplanted is alive, thinks, is conscious. How do I do that?"[45] The EEG wasn't enough. The graphs showing auditory stimulation weren't enough. As he leaned back into his first-class seat, the engines whining to life beneath the plane, White knew that *none* of the fancy advances in technology in the West were enough to show that a disembodied brain was thinking. No. He needed to go backward to move forward. The answer had been in the past all along—not in Demikhov's heart and lung transplants, not in his ventricle work and revascularization, but with the very publicity stunt that had first set White's mind spinning.

Demikhov had shown the puppy's second head drinking milk to demonstrate that it was still alive. You needed a face to do that. The solution wasn't more isolated brains—it was to transplant the head itself, with all its nerves intact. White would go back to the drawing board and design an operation—no, *two* operations. Monkey A and Monkey B, side by side. And he'd take another lesson from Demikhov as well: if he was going to do groundbreaking work, he might as well do it in public.

*Chapter 5*

# FRANKENSTEIN'S MONKEY

*A*utumn *light diffused through clouded glass and into the Brain Research Lab.* The sun was setting, though it was not quite five in the afternoon. Maurice Albin and Robert White ought to have been headed home, but they awaited a guest: Oriana Fallaci.

At thirty-eight years old, the Italian journalist had already been a member of the resistance during World War II and was one of a handful of daring female war journalists; her later interviews included the likes of Henry Kissinger, North Vietnamese general Võ Nguyên Giáp, and Gandhi. Even so, the attractive woman with straight blond hair and Lauren Bacall looks appeared more than a decade younger than the forty-one-year-old White—and said so, though she complimented his "sturdy" frame. She also called him "jolly."[1] Granted, White's scant remaining hair had prematurely grayed, but he'd lost the extra weight again, so it wasn't a reference to Saint Nick so much as her surprise at White's ready humor. But Fallaci hadn't come to do a puff piece; she'd come to document one of White's monkey brain isolations, which had carried on without pause since his return from Moscow the year before.

"Are you sorry you kill so many monkeys?" Fallaci asked him.

"Sure I am," White replied. "Death always disturbs me. My work isn't to bring death. It is to preserve life."[2]

The words bear strange resemblance to those uttered by White's favorite tragic hero. Victor Frankenstein begins his narrative by exclaiming that "To examine the causes of life, we must first have recourse to death," that to stall the corruption of the blooming cheek meant hours in the charnel house, picking through bones, and at the anatomy table. For White, it meant three hundred monkey heads frozen or floating in alcohol still stored in the lab, along with the brains of as many mice and no shortage of dogs. Yes, that many brains seemed like a lot. Yes, he thought they were all necessary.

He'd come a long way from that first isolation; the surgery taking place at eight o'clock the next morning would be performed "hot"— that is, without the cooling of the brain that had once seemed so necessary. White had been perfecting his revascularization techniques, moving quickly the way Demikhov had done, using speed and precision to isolate the brain and keep it working at optimal temperature. Would Fallaci understand that? Maybe, maybe not. He led her to where his little "patients" were kept, in a separate room where the vet technicians kept them reasonably clean and fed.

The monkey for the next morning's surgery dined on orange, banana, and pellets of chow with suitable vitamins. Albin and the veterinarians on staff would be giving the monkey a thorough physical to make sure of good health. Fallaci asked the monkey's name, but the monkey didn't have one. Could *she* name it? Albin didn't see why not, so the journalist called him Libby. (She mistook him for a female because the macaque was quite small.) Introductions over, the team shut the lab down for the night, leaving a resident to keep an eye on things. Surgery would begin the next morning, bright and early.

White said good night to Fallaci and headed home to a late supper. Having a journalist in the lab had not been to everyone's taste, particularly not the more reserved members of staff—but this time, it wasn't even White's idea. Fallaci had contacted him through channels at the university; he'd originally thought it was for a student research report. White would have to admit, however, that the inquiry flattered him. Demikhov had appeared in *Life*; now White's work would turn up in *Look*, the weekly's chief competitor. Their labor would reach hundreds. A little publicity couldn't hurt, could it?

By the time White scrubbed in the next morning, Albin had already anesthetized the monkey and shaved it, too. Leo Massopust, a neurophysiologist who'd joined the team, would be monitoring the patient's brain waves throughout the surgery, a role more important now than before because the uncooled brain was in a more delicately sensitive state. White clenched his surgery pipe between his teeth and entered a surprisingly crowded lab. There'd been a few changes in staff of late. Albin and Verdura were still there, joined by experimental psychologist Lee Wolin, as well as Satoru Kadoya, already a pioneer in spine surgery; White's new assistant, David Yashon; and the eager Italian journalist.

"Coffee and donuts are coming," White said. His secretary, also named Patty, brought them in moments later, just as Albin was inserting a tube into the monkey's femoral artery. White peered at Fallaci over his mug. "The brain of a monkey isn't so different from that of a man," he offered. She wrote that down. "The procedure for isolating a human brain would be about the same, except in terms of scale." She wrote *that* down, too.[3] Then Albin indicated that they were ready, and White stepped into position, and into focus. Oriana Fallaci became part of the background while he worked, all but forgotten as White did what he did best—smoking, joking, and discussing the news as his fingers worked swift and certain. Fallaci would later call them pianist's fingers and priest's hands, and describe their movements as a perfect dance, entirely divorced from White's innocuous chatter. She didn't know him the way Albin did. White's team knew that every muscle in White's body was on fire; it was exhausting work—and hot work, too, since they used a cautery blade to cut and stop blood flow simultaneously by burning and sealing tissue. White's glasses clouded, but he didn't stop until the skull was finally naked of flesh. Fallaci appeared at his elbow.

"Would you call this animal alive?" she asked, pointing to the admittedly bizarre half-flesh, half-skeletal macaque. White studied the monitors. Pressure, temperature, brain waves—everything checked out. "Why not?" he shot back. It wasn't time for conversation. He had yet to do the most difficult part. The blood feeding the brain came from four major vessels, the right and left common carotid arteries and the right and left vertebral arteries. Without the aid of supercooling, White had to ligate the arteries (that is, tie them off), snip them, insert them into a T-cannula, ligate and snip and insert the same vessels from the larger monkey, and then restore flow—in *under three minutes*. *That* was the real story here, and he wanted the journalist to focus on it. He beckoned Fallaci to follow him as Albin administered another dose of anesthetic to keep the monkey under. "You must understand," he said, wiping his glasses. The sensation wasn't in the optics, but in the nearly invisible switch he and his team were about to make. This wasn't about bodies; it was all about the brain.[4] The *living* brain. White signaled that they were ready for the donor monkey; it was time to do the real work.

The donor frightened Fallaci—or at least, she'd call him "frightening." And well she might: scar-ridden and aggressive, he didn't play well with other monkeys, biting and scratching. He cared much less for his handlers. Once they had him anesthetized, they turned the recipient, Libby, onto his stomach. White hovered over the small macaque's arteries, ready to begin. Massopust confirmed that the signals were good and Albin nodded. They had done this before. Over a hundred surgeries had failed, but twice as many had succeeded. Failing today, however, would be failing publicly.

The mood sizzled like high-tension wires; White set his pipe aside and everyone went silent. Fallaci was about to witness the *other* side of a White Surgery, the hyperfocus of a man who knew seconds meant lives. White used a curved needle to hook and tie the four arteries, and then liberated the head from everything else. Ligate recipient, T-cannula, ligate donor. "Open the line," he said.[5] Blood flowed from the larger monkey, and White severed the last connection between the smaller monkey's brain and its own body. Everyone watched the monitors. There was a blip. Then the brain waves picked up, even more vigorously than before. White breathed a sigh of relief. Blood flow had been reestablished without any loss of function, at regular temperature. He went through the rest of the work at his ease, removing the bony casing so the bright orange bulb of brain stood alone. He showed it to the journalist. This was one for the papers.

White kept the brain going till nine in the evening, putting it through a series of tests measuring metabolic rate, pressure, and response to stimuli. Team members leaned on tables, propped up by coffee and stale pastry. They'd all had enough. They needed sleep and decent meals, so White cut the connections and watched as the monkey's brain function slowly dipped in register from peaks to flat line. "Can you hold it for the photo?" Fallaci asked—and so he did, cupping it between his palms. Fallaci asked if it was now mere tissue;

White shook his head. "It's much more. It was perfume, and now it's an empty bottle," he said, "but the fragrance is still there."[6] A fitting end, he thought. But he had other work to do, and anyway, it was nearly Saturday—his day with his tribe of children, taking the grocery store by storm and collecting calves' brains from the butcher shop.

Oriana Fallaci was used to being told when the interview had ended. She was just as used to ignoring it. "Dr. White," she asked, and her tone seemed sharper than before, "do you fear the extreme consequences of your work?" White chuckled. Did she mean Aldous Huxley, *Brave New World?* The question seemed naive, out of character with everything White had shown her—all his careful preparations, his methodical steps. Of course he'd thought of the possibilities of his work; he'd thought of nothing else—the whole point was to save lives. Hadn't he said so?

Science was always aware of the dangers, he told her, "But being able to accomplish certain things doesn't mean that we will accomplish them."[7] That was, he assured her, the whole point of scientific ethics. And anyway, what she'd witnessed today was principally about how to keep a (monkey) brain alive, how to study its functions independent of the body—not about whether such surgery was right to perform on humans. "Ah, but you said it *could* be done in humans," Fallaci reminded him. Perhaps he had let that slip. "Yes, today, we could keep Einstein's brain alive," White agreed. But that didn't mean it ought to be done, or that he was recommending it.[8] She persisted, however, pressing the question about whether that brain would still *be* Einstein. What is a brain without its body, after all?

Fallaci had managed the turn of the screw, engaging White in one of his favorite subjects, the one about which he was most gregarious: the possibilities of a bodiless mind. "When I detach the brain from the body, the intelligence and personality remain intact," White assured her. He went so far as to suggest that the personality was inborn, present in the embryo, revealing much of his Catholic predilections but ignoring contemporary debates about nature vs. nurture and the continual development of connections in the brain as we age. He didn't stop there. He told her that a bodiless brain would have so little else to trouble it, it might act as a supercomputer would. Mathematical problems, ethical problems, all might be entirely simpler to solve for a brain lacking external stimuli.[9] Could we save people by transplanting their brains? Well, no, because reattaching the nerves would be much too difficult. Could we save them by transplanting the whole head? Yes, in theory, though White admitted even he himself was a little horrified by the thought of people walking about with mismatched heads and bodies. No, we aren't ready; we have to stick with monkeys and dogs for now. Human experiment must come later, after we have had a chance to consider the matter from ethical and religious perspectives. Fallaci smiled in her demure way. "So it's a moral problem we have to face," she said.[10]

A moral problem. White caught the bus from his lab and settled into the nearest seat. Probably he thought in retrospect, *I went a bit too far*. Theology was based on scientific theories now long outdated, even he admitted that. For centuries, doctors had said that death comes when the heart stops and the patient stops breathing. But they were wrong. Death comes three to five minutes later, when the brain gives up the ghost. Sometimes brain death precedes the death of the body, such as when the brain has died and the body still breathes on machines. White watched dreary streets slide by the frosted pane. At that very moment, a beautiful and intelligent young girl—a pianist, only eighteen years old—lay in his hospital, desperate for a kidney. But White couldn't give one to her. And he couldn't pluck one from a paralyzed or comatose donor of the same blood type, even if he'd had one handy.[11]

He'd told Fallaci as much. Neither legal nor religious principles had quite caught up to science. And then she'd asked the question that most troubled him: "Do you mean the entire concept of life needs to be defined again?"[12]

Yes, he told her. Emphatically, unapologetically yes. Death is a dead brain. And a live brain is alive. How much clearer could he put it? "If I cut off your arms and legs, if I cut out your tongue"—all things, admittedly, he'd just done to Libby—then even with blinded eyes, new lungs, and a new heart, she would remain the same individual. "But," he continued, "if I take your brain, nothing remains of you."[13] He'd said that before to Maurice Albin, to Javier Verdura, to his wife, Patricia; he had even spoken of it to theologians and to his own priest at Our Lady of Peace. "What is the soul?" was a question White asked himself every time he held in his hands that amorphous bundle of jelly and nerves, so unremarkable—so unlike what the Russians had hoped for when they studied the brain of the genius and the fool. Under the microscope, the tissues all look the same, and yet something special, something unique and strange, unbridled and individual, lived there. "The soul," he told Fallaci, "is *in* the brain."[14]

Then Fallaci had asked her final, killer question: Doesn't that mean the monkey has a soul, just as you do?

"No," he told her. It did not. And that was that.

White stood up at his bus stop and ambled down the aisle. "Good night, Doc!" the driver called cheerily.

"Night." White smiled back. What was there to worry about, after all? An attractive young lady had matched him wit for wit; he'd enjoyed it, even. A first real taste of publicity, that's all it was. What was the harm in that? White went home to his supper, as he had the night before. And as before, the attractive young lady went back to her hotel to write copy.

## SOUL SEARCHING

"Libby had eaten her last meal," began Fallaci's article. The monkey's eyes "were so sad, so defenseless," with hands like "those of a newly born child."[15] At every opportunity, Fallaci reminded the reader of the monkey's personality, humanizing the creature, and (partly by naming it) giving the monkey center stage. She described White as possessed of a mysterious joy, with a gleam in his eye as he approached the "blasphemous challenge." Not all of her epithets were negative; she likened White to a NASA engineer launching a rocket (entirely appropriate, more so than she knew) and praised his acumen. But she also described Libby's discarded body lying lifeless on the floor. She talked about the animal's brain, too: "All Libby had been, her joys and fears, her reactions and memories, the jungle in which she had been born, the net in which she had been captured, the cage in which she had been imprisoned . . . everything was still living inside that brain without flesh."[16] What would happen when the brain awoke? she asked. Would it be aware of the nothingness it had become?

White had worked hard to ensure that the brain continued to think, but in Fallaci's account, his triumph echoes with disembodied horror, with White himself presented as a Frankenstein figure, focused so narrowly on the *can* that he had not engaged with the *should*. Oriana Fallaci's profile of Robert White would become, in a way, the most powerful expression of White's work ever written, not because it provided the best scientific account, nor even because of its wide readership, but because of its insistence on grappling with those "extreme *consequences*," those thrilling shadows pulsing with possibility . . . and because Fallaci had no interest in taking White's word for what was appropriate or necessary.

"The Dead Body and the Living Brain" appeared on November 28,

1967, not with the power of an atom bomb but with the timed fuse of consecutive explosions. It was but the latest article of its kind in an increasingly bitter contest between science and animal rights, all playing out in the public arena. *Life* magazine had once carried the story of Demikhov's two-headed dog; in 1966, it ran a very different kind of narrative: "Concentration Camp for Dogs." A distressing animal trade had developed in the United States, the article claimed, one that stole family pets from backyards and auctioned them to major research institutions. The feature included a photo of Lancer, a mixed-breed mongrel who'd escaped a lab and made the long journey home to his family wearing a tag reading "H.M.S."—Harvard Medical School.[17] The highest institution in the nation was apparently sending its graduate students out in unmarked vans to "sweep" the streets of loose animals. Another article, this one in *Sports Illustrated*, presented the sordid tale of a dealer-to-lab trade, complete with horror stories of dogs piled on top of one another and shipped overland.[18] The first article connected research labs to World War II concentration camps, a horror still fresh in the minds of many; the second likened them to slave ships.*

These efforts had resulted in the US Animal Welfare Act (AWA) of 1966, signed by President Lyndon B. Johnson. The law put at least some regulation on how animals could be treated in labs, but it was a beginning, not an end. A new battleground had opened, not over dogs, but over nonhuman primates, helped along by Jane Goodall's popular work with chimpanzees. Earlier in the decade, she'd first reported their use of tools, an aptitude once thought to be distinctive to humans. If "sentience" refers to a creature's cognitive ability and "proximity" to

---

*Lesley Sharp, an anthropologist and author of *Animal Ethos*, has done an interesting comparison of the different types of persuasive photojournalism accounts from this era, noting the way each sets an innocent public against nefarious research establishments using the dog—man's best friend—as an emotional icon.

a creature's sameness to us, then taken together, the very things that made the chimp or macaque most useful in experimental science also made it closest to human, to humanity.[19] Goodall's findings begged the question: If we were unwilling to experiment on dogs, how could we experiment on our nearer "cousins"? And what was the point of isolating a monkey's brain, anyway? Or any brain? Was it needed?

For that, White had a very clear and specific answer: yes. You weren't going to sort out diseases like Alzheimer's without understanding basic brain chemistry.[20] But of course, that wasn't really what Fallaci was getting at. She had talked White into a corner—and that was hard to do. White would later complain that Fallaci had twisted his words, that she'd asked questions about monkey souls and then "answered them herself."[21] (Henry Kissinger would say something very similar— or rather, he would complain that his interview with her was "the most disastrous encounter he'd ever had with a member of the press," while conceding that the substance of her piece was more or less accurate.)[22]

Fallaci was not an animal rights activist. She had no dealings with the Friends of Animals groups that would later coalesce around PETA. Instead, her aims were almost always to *unsettle*. "To me, being a journalist means being disobedient," she once wrote. "And being disobedient means being in opposition. In order to be in opposition, you have to tell the truth. And the truth is always the opposite of what people say."[23] The questions she had asked White during the surgery, and then the next day when she pursued him (uninvited) into his lab, didn't unsettle him; he loved to be provocative. But presented in print, with context excised away like monkey flesh from a gleaming skull, the interview appeared to reveal inconsistencies. Blind spots. Moral gaps. White frowned over the article, but he kept it. Several copies of it, in fact.

The most troubling thing to White wasn't Fallaci's distortion of the monkey's plight, or even her intentional sensationalism. What bothered him was the accusation that White had not thought through the philosophical implications of his work; she had tried to catch him out, tried to show that his theology had gone wrong. Fallaci's article made it sound like monkeys had souls.

The Greek philosopher Plato called the "I" outside the body the "soul." Catholic Christianity proclaimed much the same. A living being sits at the unification, the soldered joint of body and soul. Separate them, and you might free the soul, but you do so through the death of the body. As a surgeon, White worked every day at that crucial intersection. Once, he operated on the brain of a man he knew well. The man died, and in White's hand, the brain he had once been was reduced to a ball of jelly: "All his good and evil, all his personality was inside this piece of tissue," but now, they were no more.[24] Where had his spark of being come from? Where did it go? Whatever the answers, the brain, White was certain, was the essence, the self, the soul.

This may not sound revolutionary. Many adherents of Western religions share White's faith in the immortal soul. But White was also playing with fire. By saying the human brain was the "self," he was also claiming it as the seat of *life*, the animating principle. As a generic philosophical sentiment, a living isolated brain or soul seems perfectly benign. But considered instead as a physical object to cut with a scalpel, separating brain from body meant deciding where life begins, and where it ends. "It sounds Frankensteinian, it sounds too far out," White would admit.[25] But he had never seen *Frankenstein* entirely as a cautionary tale. "We're on the edge," White would tell *People* magazine a few years later, "much as we were before Einstein came along and made that quantum jump from Newtonian physics."[26] This time, he would be Einstein.

The way forward lay with cephalic transplantation: the true

transplant of one head onto another body, all sutures connected, all life supported, a composite being. Only then could he prove that the spikes on electrograph paper represented not the mere electrical mood swings of an unknowable glob of tissue, but instead the living thoughts of a living thing. The brain. The sole part of the body where, as White said again and again, "the human spirit and soul reside."[27]

The *human* spirit. White's chief complaint against Fallaci would be that the journalist put words in his mouth about monkeys and souls. But monkeys didn't have souls; Catholic doctrine had been pretty firm about that. What they had was . . . hard to define. Animals weren't considered material beings. They weren't rational, had no concept of wrong and right. Their "souls" were just the principle of life, of matter. A single cell of bacteria was alive, tumors were alive, trees were alive; none of them even had brains, and none had a *spiritual* soul.[28] "The soul of brutes," went the doctrine, "can only exist in matter," and when that matter dies, so dies the soul.[29] They were not immortal. And yet when successfully operated on, Libby and his fellow (un)lucky primates outlived their own bodies. If not a soul, what winked on and off in those suspended brains?

Fallaci had proved an extremely effective antagonist, and White never forgot it—sometimes eschewing the timeline and suggesting that Fallaci's article had helped "put together all the various pieces that became PETA."[30] He lay at her feet the beginnings of a very different kind of publicity, and of the nickname he would soon acquire among his critics: Dr. Butcher. But he didn't capitulate, either. He didn't stop working toward his dream.

Two years went by. White had not been idle in his other roles as surgeon, professor, and head of the BRL. His hospital neurosurgery department grew, and students under White's tutelage at the university—now known as Case Western—often did residencies with him at Metro. Among them was Norman Taslitz, an MD/PhD who came on board as White was carefully finalizing his method for a new type of transplant surgery. The clock was ticking and the decade running out, but no matter. Fallaci had claimed in her article that Libby's isolation was the most extraordinary surgery ever performed. But the real Frankenstein moment had only just arrived.

## HEAD A, MONKEY B

"Can we go play with the monkeys?"

Another Saturday had come, this one in late February 1970. Richard Nixon was one year into his first term as president, and Simon & Garfunkel's "Bridge over Troubled Water" was in its first of six weeks at the top of the charts. The morning was bitter cold, though the mercury managed to reach almost 50 degrees Fahrenheit during the day. White piled the older children into the family station wagon; Michael, fourth born, fought for the front seat.[31] They were off to visit Dad's office.

For a ten-year-old, the Metro lab might as well have been magical, a science fiction space station and mystery theater in one. Michael had once gained permission to take a monkey brain to school for show-and-tell, a stunt that didn't go over particularly well with his teacher, though it no doubt won him temporary fame among his fellow third graders. Once inside the laboratory parking lot, the children bounced out of the wood-paneled wagon and into the well-known corridors. All sorts of animals could be seen in their respective cages along the wall, some with thin wires protruding from their heads like antennae. Research, said the adults, but for the White clan, these were playmates. They'd recently had a lopsided kitten as a pet; White had removed one hemisphere of its brain to test the cat's reactions. She walked sideways, earning her the nickname Sidewinder.[32] All very well, of course, but the main attraction for Michael and the others was the monkeys.

These weren't just any primates—White called them the PhD monkeys. Neurophysiologist Leo Massopust and psychologist Lee Wolin had begun training a group of adult rhesus macaques to pass a series of six tests intended to measure cognitive function: perception, thinking, reasoning, and remembering.[33] They were trained to do a series of activities for food rewards: pulling levers, pressing buttons, choosing images or colors . . . The complexity of the tasks required more than six months of work with each monkey.

"They bite, be careful," White cautioned as the children pulled faces at the cages and offered the monkeys treats. Even the best-trained macaques were bad tempered; they had a reputation for being territorial, violent, mean. Science writer Deborah Blum's *The Monkey Wars* describes the apparent paradox of rhesus macaques' reputation as the perfect research monkey; on the one hand, they're strong and resilient, the "street toughs of the monkey world," meaning they survive and remain hardy despite lab conditions.[34] On the other hand, however, their independence means they're never truly domesticated, not even when born and raised in captivity. White's macaques bit their caretakers, they bit one another,* and they would have no qualms about biting the child of the imperious surgeon they'd learned to despise. Social, intense, frustrated by boredom, physically strong, and untamable, the "trouble" with macaques also offered their greatest strength: people tended not to get attached to them. And yet they had the intelligence of a four-year-old human—the age of young Richard, White's eighth child—making them intellectually *more* developed than either Marguerite or Ruth, the youngest and last of the clan at three and one years old, respectively. A

---

*They have a rather disturbing habit of biting one another's penises off.

smart monkey could perform tasks, have its brain altered, and perform them again. Using macaques, White and his team had proven the last piece of his perfusion work: freezing the brain (dropping it below 15 degrees Celsius) did not result in a loss of cognition. The monkeys, rewarmed, performed the tests as well as before, offering a bridge from nonhuman primate to human testing.[35] White didn't know it then, but this technique would go on to save decades of cardiac arrest victims. Heart attack sometimes leads to brain damage, as the weakened heart can't pump enough blood; cooling the brain means it doesn't need as much oxygen, buying surgeons precious time to unblock a patient's arteries. Preserving the life of the human brain was the end goal of everything White did in the lab—every surgery, every experiment. Even this next one.

White traced a chalk line on the floor of the lab. It looked like a dance pattern. He had planned it out, literally step by step, with Verdura, Massopust, Wolin, and Taslitz. He had painstakingly outlined the footwork for each participant, complete with arrows to indicate which direction they should travel. To the untrained eye, a chaotic shuffling of tick marks; to White, the choreography of more than thirty highly skilled professionals—surgeons, anesthesiologists, nurses, animal technicians, and monitoring scientists. The sequence had been perfected over the course of months, and a series of dry runs on eight small rhesus monkeys; White didn't isolate the brains in these trials, though—he no longer needed to. Instead, his team practiced carefully removing the monkey's head from its shoulders while keeping the vascular system intact.

The carotid-jugular circulation was interrupted at the base of the head and the top of the neck, the monkey's own arteries elongated by a series of four coiled loops of tubing. The trachea and esophagus were then severed, and an incision made between the fourth and sixth cervical vertebrae, known as a cervical laminectomy.[36] A schematic drawing demonstrated the outcome: the monkey's head buoyed above its body, resting on the coils of tubing as if upon a ruffled collar. White called these efforts "the preparations," but the trials did not create headless monkeys; rather, they created monkeys whose heads had become somewhat remote from their bodies.[37] The surgeries mimicked certain kinds of trauma that occur in car accidents, where the skull becomes detached from the spinal column and the nerves severed, but with one unusual addition: the tubing could be uncoiled, stretched out, and the head moved even farther away from its body.

"One of the heads woke up while I was on duty," Taslitz told White one morning after his overnight shift.[38] It was terrifying, he admitted, like a horror movie—alone in the dark with the monkey head staring at him. *Well, there's still a lot we don't know about the brain*, White said, seemingly unsurprised. In spite of extensive research, it still offered the greatest enigma, the greatest challenge. "Since the beginning of human existence the entirety of what man has accomplished," he'd later write, "is the result of the activity of this most complex and unique object in the known world": the brains of humans.[39] The brains of monkeys, too.

White watched his children playing with the primates, aware that two Saturdays hence, the lab would be a sea of people following the chalk lines. Room to work would be in seriously short supply. There would be two monkeys, not one. Both would need to be separated from their bodies and tethered by their arteries and veins, their breathing aided by machines, and their blood pressure, EEG, cerebral fluid, metabolic rate, and temperature monitored. It would be hot, strenuous, elbow-bumping activity. And if their previous work was anything to go by, it would take hours and hours to complete—with no ability to stop between procedures, no chance to rest. Cross-sections and drawings, notes and scribbles, methods and plans papered over White's desk; *head*

*A, body B.* White didn't call it a head transplant. He called it a body transplant. They were going to give the organs of one primate to the brain of another, all at once. And while Oriana Fallaci might question whether such actions were necessary, White believed all of his work offered a chance at saving future lives.

White had seen so many minds lost, damaged, locked in endless coma—children who never spoke again, lovers who never embraced again. A year earlier, a seventeen-year-old gymnast living in the area had been working out on a trampoline. A moment's inattention, and he fell on his head. His name was Peter, and he knew immediately that his neck was broken. With surprising calm, he asked the arriving paramedics not to move his head too much.[40] White met with Peter's frightened parents and asked them for permission to cool his spine. They wanted to know (rightly) if it had ever been done before. It had—on monkeys, on the "Libbys" of the Brain Research Lab's primate-laden cages. The parents consented, and Peter was sedated on White's operating table to be perfused in hopes of halting the nerve damage. Hours later, he awoke. Within weeks, he'd regained some use of his arms—and even of his hands. Peter M. Sikora went on to become a judge in Cuyahoga County, Ohio, because of a monkey and a surgeon and a calculated risk.

If the fight with Fallaci had given White pause, his doubts evaporated in the heat of lived experience. For White, the ends justified the means. "Let's say a man comes before you," White would tell London's *Sunday Telegraph* in coming years, "totally paralyzed from the neck down" and facing organ failure.[41] "Are you going to sit there and tell him he can't have a transplant?" And what was a kidney or a heart compared to a whole body, with all of its systems working? Until now, it had all been hypothetical. "I am not really interested in human head transplants," he'd told Fallaci during their interview. It just wasn't true.

·    ·    ·

March 14, 1970. The weather in Shaker Heights had turned cold again, down into the twenties with occasional flurries dusting the panes. White woke extra early, well before the rest of the family, and wandered downstairs among the leafy green of children's Saint Patrick's Day crafts. Patricia was Boston Irish, after all, her ancestors the Toland sisters, two of the four thousand Irish Famine orphans who were sent to Australia as indentured servants.[42] Corned beef and soda bread would be on the hob all day on Saint Pat's, and White, who once won "Irishman of the Year" at the downtown Cleveland celebration, would take his green-clad children to the parade. He wasn't thinking about any of that today, though. He tucked his surgery pipe into the pocket of his winter coat and headed out in the cold and dark. It would be a Saturday to remember.

At the lab, the coffee pots were full and hot. White tugged a towel around his neck—he'd need it for dabbing the sweat of surgery—and adjusted his square black frames. Just like before, he reminded the men; the first steps, at least, would be the same as with the coil-necked preparations. Except now, of course, it mattered more. The teams took their places: two sets of surgeons, two sets of other vital staff, in two different operating rooms. The monkeys had been shaved and marked; a literal "A" had been written on the head of one in permanent marker, a "B" on the body of the second. The sound of exhales could be heard as team members' nerves escaped under pressure. White set his pipe aside and checked the time on the large IBM clockface above them. "Stand by," he said, allowing Albin to administer a dose of anesthetic—20 milligrams per kilogram of body weight at regular intervals. The teams, synchronized to the clocks in either room, put tubes in the tracheas of both monkeys, each attached to its own Mark 8 ventilator. The green-and-red device of semitransparent plastic set the flow rate for oxygen. *Ticktock*; it was time to make the first incision.

White and his team cut a circle through the soft tissue, the full circumference about the neck of the monkey who was to donate its head. Deeper and deeper they went, carefully separating the delicate arteries and veins and dividing the tissue around the cervical vertebra.[43] White had to trust that all was going according to plan in the second operating room, that the other team, working under Verdura, was watching the clock just as he was to coordinate their efforts. Ten minutes, twenty, half an hour, an hour; slowly the interior of the neck was exposed, and the trachea and esophagus could be severed. White checked the monitors; machines managed respiration, in-out, as the chest cavity filled with oxygen. He made the cut. A few moments more and White arrived at last at the spinal cord. "Prepare the catecholamine," White told his nurse. The drug would counteract spinal shock, wherein reflex, motor, and sensory function would be lost below the injury site. He divided the cord, and the nurse injected—next he would cauterize the vertebral sinus, a vein that runs through the spine.[44] Once complete, he could completely transect the spinal column. A few patient strokes of the cautery blade, and the head and body were severed—all except for the neurovascular bundles. All these vessels were ligated, tied off one by one. Surgeons and nurses held their breath; each vessel needed to be cut and reattached in microseconds. A wrong move, and the monkey would bleed out. White gave the signal, and in a matter of minutes the vessels had been cannulated, attached to coiled tubes, and plugged back into their severed ends. The monkey's head rested just above its body like the dangling receiver on a corded telephone. White and his team had come as far as ever they had. This had been their previous stopping point, a place they knew—a comfort zone of sorts. What they prepared to do next had never been done before.

Down the hall, the sound of wheels on polished tile announced the arrival of Monkey B. The second team, sweat-stained and breathless, pushed the mobile operating table into place on the floor's chalk lines. The already warm room became almost steamy with the sudden doubling of human and monkey bodies, amid a tangle of wires and tubes, fluid and respiration lines. Hands reached over one another, bodies twisted at awkward angles as they attempted to get purchase on their respective subjects. The blood flow from the body of Monkey B needed to be transferred now to Monkey A's head. In many ways, it was the perfection of White's early use of the monkey "blood bag." Before, an intact monkey had supported a disembodied brain; now the head and body would be united. The chatter so common in White's operating room dropped to a low hum. It was not like the movies.

In the classic Boris Karloff *Frankenstein* film, a careless assistant collects a bodiless brain from a lab—a floating repository of self, ready to be plugged into any available body. White claimed to love the part where Fritz (Igor in later renditions) drops the brain on the floor, and so must choose an abnormal brain to replace it. In reality, neither brain would have been of any use; they had been robbed of precious lifeblood for too long. White and his team could not simply remove Monkey B's head all at once and replace it with that of Monkey A. No; what ensued over the next few hours was the careful *weaving together* of the two creatures. Each time they disconnected one stream of that vital fluid from Body B, it had to be reattached at the same junction on Head A. As each plastic tube from B fed A, a little more of B's own brain died. As each vessel from Head A was supplanted by Body B, a little more of A's body died. They were becoming a composite being, a man-made conjoined twin not so unlike Demikhov's dogs, though far more advanced. Partway through the surgery, the EEG signals of B slowed to a stop, a gradual decline of blips as blood ebbed away. Head A, still deeply under anesthetic, continued to generate brain waves.

"We're all right," White said, peering at a wall of dials behind him, "we're okay."[45] The towel around his neck was soaked, and he reached for a sip of cold coffee as they waited for the blood flow to stabilize. The clock above now registered well past midday, but no one was counting anymore. The technicians gave the all clear; Head A now fed entirely from Body B. It was time to cut away the last vestiges of Body A, removing the head from its spine. A few snips more, and the dislocation was complete; White's nurses discarded Body A and Head B. Body B and Head A awaited their final stages as a new creature, one not quite finished.

White directed the nurses to administer anticoagulant, necessary until they could attach vein to vein and be rid of the tubing. He had them administer antibiotics, too, to ward off infection, just in case.[46] It was time, at last, to bring the head and body fully together—to remove the tubes, suture the vessels, screw plates to the bony nubs of vertebrae, and close the muscle tissue and skin around the wound. Anxious eyes watched the dashboard of measurement devices; it was the third time in hours they'd had to open and close arteries and veins, the third time they had to wait to see if circulation would return. When they were finished, the monkey stared, gap-mouthed, at the ceiling; it no longer appeared to be part of some butchery, but rather a single monkey with a circular set of stitches around its neck. Brain waves kept on. Circulation returned. But still the monkey remained an empty vessel—a useless blank. White stepped away from the table and picked up his discarded pipe. Now they had to wait for the monkey to wake up. *If* it woke up.

The procedure had taken a total of eighteen hours.[47] The surgeons were exhausted and cramped from standing hunched around their tables; the nurses, technicians, and others monitoring the vitals blinked bleary eyes. White sat in a nearby chair, eyes watering behind fogged lenses, one hand resting on the bowl of his pipe. "Another fifteen or sixteen minutes" and the anesthesia should wear off, he thought.[48] The monkey would wake. At least he *hoped* it would. To send them all home with no better achievement than a monkey in a coma would not do at all. Then, the first signs: "Doc, look here!" Satoru Kadoya had been monitoring the monkey's vitals, and he'd seen an eyelid flutter. Sore muscles forgotten, White sprang up and peered over the table. First one eye, then the other. Then the faintest twitch of the lips, a smacking, the movement of the tongue.[49] Bit by bit, the creature swam toward consciousness, and suddenly, its eyes were open and tracking. White tapped its nose gently with a pair of forceps, and the monkey attempted to bite him. For a moment, all was shocked silence. Then the operating room erupted in cheers. Several team members danced; one of them screamed. They brought a pencil and let the monkey chew it, then tapped its cheeks and watched it blink, fed it ice and hunted for useful stimuli . . . The vocal box nerves—along with the nerves leading to the lower body—had been severed with the spine. Paralyzed from the neck down, awake and alive on the top of a foreign body, the macaque was, in White's own words, "dangerous, pugnacious, and very unhappy."[50] But it was also *alive*.

That knowledge roused White and carried him through the rest of the day; everything he'd worked so hard to prove had come to fruition. The creature in his laboratory was in every way a monkey—the *same* monkey. It certainly seemed to remember White, if only to hate him. "What have I done?" he wondered. "Have I reached a point where the human soul can be transplanted? And if so, what does that mean?"[51]

On his way home to the warmth of his Shaker Heights study, White had decided that what could be done for the monkey could be done for man.[52] But to do so would take convincing whole disciplines—whole populations—that life needed to be defined afresh. Say what he would about life being housed in the brain, there was as yet no official statement from either medicine or religion about *when life ended*. And no one would let him go further, not even one step, without a decision here. Monkey A lived on; he would make it for almost nine days before the body rejected the head. But Monkey B? He was gone. Could you transplant a human head onto a brain-dead body? Of course you could. But a brain-dead body was living tissue, and if you thought of living tissue as a living being—well. Frankenstein may have built his monster from cadavers, but White needed living parts. And unless some very important changes happened, the question haunting his next endeavor wouldn't be about animal experiments. It might very well be about human murder.

White kept a plastic replica of the human brain on his desk. People would later ask (some already did), "What are you doing all this for?" Why do it, why bother? To take a body and give it to a brain, wouldn't that be selfish somehow? All those organs going to only one recipient? But then, they had never sat with the parents of a dying child, had they? They had never sat on committees with the responsibility of approving organs for transplant.[53] There were bodies out there. He knew already of those in Russia, the ones Demikhov had spoken of, warehoused in hospitals in Moscow, in Kiev; he'd been invited back to the country— he was planning to go. But brain death occurred everywhere; every nation had its share of beating-heart bodies with empty brains. What if Frankenstein was right, and "Literature has run ahead of us"?[54] It was time to catch up—not just the science, but the Catholic doctrine, too. There were ways to evolve that. There had to be.

Chapter *6*

# THE MODERN PROMETHEUS

Who are you? What are you? You are not in that dead body. Let's be practical. You are in the tissues of your brain, in the loci of the human spirit.

—Robert White

*Y*ou *are your brain, while yet it lives. A dead brain, floating in solution, is an in-*animate thing, bloodless and no more alive than the scalpel that cuts it into pieces. A brain suffused with blood and oxygen and sending signals to the EEG—*that* is a living and thinking brain. We can tell the living from the dead. But where is the fine and subtle line between one state and the other? When does the animating principle ... cease? "The boundaries which divide Life from Death are at best shadowy and vague," wrote Edgar Allan Poe in 1844.[1] Those boundaries would remain murky and indistinct over the next hundred and fifty years.

White's patchwork monkeys—eating, blinking, biting, and living on borrowed bodies for days—offered the first concrete proof that the mind could outlive the body. The peaks and valleys of the EEGs in White's lab weren't mistakes; these active brain waves were the very essence of life. "I thought the issue was settled," White would later confess to an interviewer from the BBC.[2] But though the monkey surgery might suggest life began and ended in the brain, it also ushered in a host of new ethical considerations. The science of transplant, still in its infancy, wasn't just about organ *recipients*. It was also about *donors*, living and dead.

When White's team performed the transplant surgery, his donor monkey, Monkey B, had to remain alive and viable up to the very moment the surgeons severed the last vital connection to its head. Cut off from blood, the donor monkey's brain died, but its body lived on to support the brain of the recipient monkey, Monkey A. Monkey B had become a *beating-heart donor* rather than a cadaver, and this had consequences for any clinical application.

By the end of the 1960s, transplant surgeons, including Joseph Murray at Peter Bent Brigham Hospital, had begun the systematic use of organs from patients they believed would never wake up.[3] Murray had, in fact, performed the first organ transplant from a *cadaver* in 1962, using the kidney of a dead body to save a living one. In a beating-heart donor, however, the organs were fresher and thus more fully functional. The donor body still urinated, still circulated blood, still metabolized nutrients. Biologically alive, but "vegetative," these donors raised two terrifying possibilities: No one wants to linger forever as an unconscious lump of meat and bone. At the same time, however, no one wants their organs to be prematurely "harvested" by transplant doctors, or their body declared dead before their time.[4] The question of what to do with a patient who was brain dead exceeded mere science; the decision had to be a *moral* one. Could doctors be trusted to know when the brain had really died? In many early transplants, surgeons would be guided only by their intuition about a potential organ donor's likely survival, even while ethical rules and regulations were being furiously debated on all sides.

"Is life a beating heart or a thinking brain?" White had asked Oriana Fallaci in his 1967 interview for *Look* magazine.[5] To him, the answer seemed obvious. But accepting that "you" are your brain privileges the brain's life over the body's. For this idea to be considered ethical at all, you had to accept that the electric signal on an EEG was the only indicator of life. But that meant you also must accept that doctors would read the EEG right in the first place, and that they wouldn't be biased toward ticking the box that allowed organs to be taken. Not surprisingly, the general public were loath to trust the harvest men.

White's first successful head transplant did not mark the completion of his life's work, but its midpoint. His question had not been "Can we make a monkey's head outlive its body?" but "Can we transplant the human soul?" Now he would have to put his mission on a frustrating pause until medicine and ethics had formed an answer to a crucial question: When had a person died enough that you could gift their body to another's brain? White couldn't yet begin adapting his monkey protocols for use on humans, but he was busy working to bring faith—and public opinion—over to his side . . .

The brain death debate had already begun; in 1968, three years before White's groundbreaking surgery, an official ad hoc committee at Harvard was formed to make sense of what death truly *was*. The furor over this definition would carry on for four years, engaging activists from both animal and civil rights and culminating in a controversial legal decision. And as usual, White soon found himself in the middle of things.

## PROMETHEUS UNBOUNDED

"Life and death are ideal bounds, which I should first break through and pour a torrent of light in our dark world," says Victor Frankenstein in a nod to the god Prometheus, who steals fire from heaven for mankind. The often-forgotten subtitle of Mary Shelley's novel gives the renegade god pride of place: *The Modern Prometheus*. But though the mystery of death might have plagued humanity since our first cognizance of temporality, the concept of *brain death* didn't get much traction until 1954, when Robert S. Schwab, a neurologist at Massachusetts General Hospital, had in his care a comatose patient suffering from a severe brain hemorrhage. Schwab asked himself a simple question: Was this patient "dead or alive?"[6] A few years earlier, and the man would have been considered dead, as he could not breathe on his own. But in the 1950s, new artificial respirators could breathe *for* a patient, even if that patient were no longer conscious, by forcing air in and out of the lungs with the aid of a bellowslike device. Mass-produced for use in hospitals (and of more importance than ever in an era of the COVID-19 pandemic), these life-support systems meant death did not necessarily take its course in the usual fashion. The end of breath no longer meant the end of life, and as technology improved, it seemed even a comatose person might be kept biologically alive indefinitely. But without reflexes, without any brain waves detected by the EEG, he would remain comatose, unresponsive, "dead" to the world around him.

Death is not a point in time, but a process—and deciding when in that process to withdraw care became a decision of conscience, one that many beyond the medical community felt compelled to comment upon.[7] In an address to an international congress of anesthesiologists in 1957, Pope Pius XII exonerated physicians who removed patients from respirators from the charge of murder, stating that life-support systems were *extraordinary means* of preserving life, when only *ordinary means* were necessary.[8] Turning off the machines would result in the death of the patient, but physicians would be passive rather than active participants in it. The pope drew the line, however, at harvesting organs from a still-living body, but declined to distinguish between brain death and bodily death. Unfortunately, neurologists couldn't agree on the difference, either. The use of organs from a beating-heart donor was by no means a foregone conclusion.

Brain death began with an irreversible coma, that much was certain. When patients suffered severe damage to the brain, such as a mutilation of necessary tissues by trauma, then their coma would be permanent. Usually a patient in this condition had already lost the ability to control their lungs, so the prognosis wasn't good for their other bodily systems. French neurologists Pierre Wertheimer and M. Jouvet described this state as "death of the nervous system," after which most patients died within five days, usually from cardiac arrest as the brain stopped being able to sufficiently send signals to the body.[9] But two other French neurologists, Pierre Mollaret and Maurice Goulon, balked at using "death of the nervous system" to describe a patient who was still in the process of dying—especially if that meant treating the patient as if they had already expired. "Do we have the right," they asked, to "pretend to know the boundary between life and death?"[10] In 1967, in South Africa, surgeon Christiaan Barnard decided that he did. His bold and risky venture would galvanize the Harvard ad hoc committee into action.

Brazen, self-assured, and a darling of the international press, Barnard was prepared to face the consequences of his actions.[11] Years earlier, incensed at Demikhov's two-headed dogs, Barnard had complained that anything Russia could do, he could do better. Now he had a chance to prove it. Following a car accident, a young woman named Denise Darvall was brought to Groote Schuur Hospital in Cape Town, South Africa. She had sustained severe fractures to the skull in the accident. There appeared to be no electrical brain activity, and Barnard tested for reflexes by pouring ice water into her ear. Determining that she was indeed brain dead, he transplanted Denise's heart into a fifty-four-year-old man—the first harvesting of a "beating" human heart into the body of another. As with so many firsts, the surgery's success was partial. The man lived through the surgery but remained ill, surviving for only eighteen days after the transplant. Nonetheless, the papers declared it a triumph.

Back in the United States, Joseph Murray watched the news with interest—and growing concern. He didn't know what Barnard's criteria had been for determining Darvall's death; what if he had been mistaken? Accusations of wrongful death would critically endanger the prospects for transplant science the world over. "We need a new definition of death," Murray wrote in a letter to his colleague Henry Beecher, then the chair of anesthesiology at Mass General. Beecher couldn't agree more. He'd already sent letters out, calling for a meeting to establish an ad hoc committee on the subject at Harvard. He hadn't realized the urgency at the time, but now the meeting couldn't come soon enough. Technological ability had just outstripped the moral— and legal—frameworks separating the living and the dead.

Beecher's committee would ultimately include an attorney, a neuroscientist, a physiologist, a professor of public health, a historian, and an ethicist, along with a coterie of surgeons like Murray. Their leading concern, Beecher explained, must be the "dying patient" and the burden prolonged vegetative comas placed upon families and overcrowded hospitals. The concept of brain death, Beecher reminded the committee, was *not* created to solve problems for transplant science, and the ad hoc committee wasn't necessarily advocating policy implications. They'd been charged with defining terms, nothing more. Murray agreed, in principle. *But*, he reminded his colleagues, patients were "stacked up in every hospital in Boston" waiting for suitable kidneys.[12] Could society really afford to lose viable organs? Barnard himself perhaps said it best: "It is infinitely better to transplant a heart than to bury it so it can be devoured by worms."[13]

By August of 1968, after in-person meetings and plenty of long-distance discussions, the committee still hadn't reached an accord about what constituted brain death—or death itself, for that matter. Instead, they agreed only to slightly expand the criteria for brain death that Robert S. Schwab had proposed a decade prior—no reflexes, no breathing, and an isoelectric (flat-line) EEG—by adding that "any organ, brain or other, that no longer functions and has no possibility of functioning is for all *practical purposes dead* [emphasis mine]."[14] The brain-dead patient was *essentially* dead. That is, he would *be* dead, he could not improve, and he would not respond to any treatment. But a prognosis of death still didn't *equal* death, and the committee didn't feel confident enough to even use the word *death* to describe what they had just defined. The published title of their report set out a narrower scope: "A Definition of Irreversible Coma." The paper would appear in the *Journal of the American Medical Association* (*JAMA*), one of the most impactful medical journals worldwide. It meant wide dissemination, and yet the report had not really said anything new. An irritated Murray crossed out "coma" and wrote "DEATH" on his copy. They had wandered into the darkness, all right, but they hadn't managed to bring much light with them.

Schwab himself pushed for something a bit more concrete. "We have to define death as cessation of heartbeat," he'd told his colleagues on the committee, because no matter what definition they chose to bring forward, it would mean nothing unless it was accepted by lawyers, medical examiners, and the public.[15] And to the public, a beating heart was a live one—no matter what a hundred beeping EEG machines might say.

Robert White, on the other hand, believed the public *could* be persuaded that life began and ended in the brain, if only they were properly informed. He had not been on the Harvard committee, but he believed, like Beecher and Murray, that death and brain death were equivalent, and that an EEG could therefore measure life and death objectively. Still, the moral question mattered. And to him, there was a critical omission in Schwab's litany of institutions that'd have to be brought around: Schwab had *not* mentioned the Church. To declare a person dead was to declare that his soul had flown—to declare him brain dead was, in the absence of a new definition, to place his soul firmly in the gray matter. To move forward with a human head transplant, White would need to convince members of his own Catholic faith that the brain, not heartbeat and breath, determined life and death. As a Catholic, he needed and wanted the Catholic Church's approval, but more to the point, he wanted the Church to be speaking truth about the body and its process to its people, to the world.

In early March of 1968, just as Murray and Beecher were gathering at Harvard, White made his way to the Catholic University of America in Washington, DC. He'd come for an extended interview with *Sign*, a national Catholic magazine. The meeting took place between the appearance of Fallaci's *Look* article and White's first successful head transplant—before, that is, he had publicly revealed his plans to transplant a human brain. The topic remained incredibly poignant all the same: Was transplant science ethical? Seated in a comfortable club chair beneath the modernist paintings in a university conference room, White faced Charles E. Curran, a renowned moral theologian. "Father," he began reverently, "I find myself beset with many problems created by new advances in medicine. I'm hoping you can provide me with some answers."[16] Curran demurred at White's performative humility. He was not, himself, a medical-moral expert; if anything, White was going to know a lot more about the subject than he would. Curran wasn't affiliated with *Sign*, either, though the article featured the discussion between them. Curran cut a somewhat controversial figure. Youthful, with an attractive, fresh face and swept-back locks, Curran publicly dissented from the Catholic view on contraception. (He supported its use; the Church did not.) As a result, he had temporarily lost his tenure appointment the year before—and was reinstated only after a student and faculty strike. He would later announce his support for same-sex unions, leading the Vatican to declare him unfit to teach Catholic theology; he would be forced to leave his position at Catholic University, ultimately seeking employment at Southern Methodist University in Texas.[17] Curran smiled at White, and assured him he was unlikely to have answers to any burning questions about organ transplant.

"Well," retorted White with a laugh, "let me try you out anyway."[18] He began with the most successful of transplant surgeries, the one he'd seen himself at Brigham. Was it permissible, in the eyes of the Church, to transplant a kidney? Curran agreed that to donate a kidney would be proper Christian charity. *But what if*, White continued, removing the kidney kills the donor? Perhaps his other kidney fails, for instance. Has anyone sinned? No, Curran assured him, no one has sinned. White sat back and puffed on his pipe. "Let me go one step further," he said, "into the operations conducted by Dr. Barnard."[19]

Barnard had been in the news again after performing another, even more controversial heart transplant the past January. This time, he had transplanted the heart of a Black man named Clive Haupt into a white patient, dentist Philip Blaiberg. In apartheid South Africa, with its still segregated facilities and rampant racial injustice, the media was enthralled; would Blaiberg mind having a "colored heart," the papers wondered. From abroad, *Ebony* magazine made a bolder point: Haupt's heart would now be allowed into segregated areas where his body had never been permitted.[20] But the controversy that interested the international medical establishment rested not with the color of the donor's skin but with his beating heart.

On New Year's Day 1968, twenty-four-year-old Haupt had suffered a subarachnoid (brain) hemorrhage while swimming. That same day, his doctor, Raymond "Bill" Hoffenberg, was asked by Barnard's transplant team to pronounce the man "dead" and confirm that his heart could be used. But Hoffenberg, like many others in the medical community, was afraid to declare death while a heartbeat remained. He refused to authorize the removal of the heart "from someone who still showed signs of life."[21] Barnard, however, worried that the heart would lose its viability if he waited until Haupt had declined far enough to be declared absolutely dead before performing the transplant.

Since many comatose patients suffer heart attacks within days, Haupt's body was a sort of time bomb. "God, Bill, what kind of heart are you going to give us?" one of the surgeons (not Barnard, though he was present) asked when Hoffenberg declined a second time in less than twenty-four hours to declare the patient dead. Everyone went home to a sleepless night, Hoffenberg perhaps most of all. When dawn came, he went to the hospital early and checked his patient one last time.[22] He convinced himself that stimulation no longer elicited the reflexes he'd seen the day before, and so finally agreed that the surgery could go ahead.

Haupt was dead because his brain was dead, White explained to Curran; the heart itself was merely meat. Surely the Church didn't think a man with a heart transplant had two souls, just because the donor heart was beating when the surgeon put it in his body. Father Curran gave a wry smile. He wouldn't be caught out that way. "I don't think a man's individuality resides in his heart or his kidneys," he said. But in response to whether Barnard had been right to make his decisions, Curran deferred. He quoted Pope Pius XII's statement from

1957 instead.[23] Though mankind should always seek to preserve life, they were only required to use "ordinary means," which the pope had defined as varying "according to circumstances of persons, places, times, and culture" but "that did not involve any grave burden for oneself or another."[24] There was no need, in other words, to keep a man in Haupt's position on life support indefinitely. Of course, according to that same broad definition, perhaps organ transplants weren't "ordinary" or necessary, either.

White had to agree that a surgeon must not "overdo it" to keep a brain-dead patient alive; questions about the right to die had sprung up with life-support systems, and White knew where he stood on the matter.[25] But wherever there remained the least spark of brain life, he would—he must—use any means necessary to sustain it. White would not give in to death, even when the patient himself begged for it. This wasn't a hypothetical situation. Back in Cleveland, a young Romanian soccer player had come to visit family over the spring holiday. Let's have a game, the relatives had said, a Sunday soccer match. Having brought his team to victory, the youth climbed atop a celebratory human pyramid. Then came the sway, a wrong step, and it toppled. He fell forward and broke his neck. Young, beautiful, dark-eyed, and with a whole life before him, the soccer star could no longer move his arms or legs or even breathe on his own. One of White's residents cared for him in the ICU and heard him whisper again and again, *"Let me die."* "Wouldn't it be better for him to pass away?" the resident asked—but White would not hear of it. "You don't let people die," he said. "You don't withdraw care. You don't quit."[26]

Across from Father Curran, White waved away the smoke that curled around his head. "The doctor wants life to continue, he wants to save it—to help it grow," he said.[27] Life mattered above all, but the question that most interested him wasn't when did life end so much as *where did it live?* That was what he wanted from the Catholic Church. "Is it so unreasonable," White asked the priest, "to assume the essence of what we mean by 'soul' resides . . . in the brain?"[28] Curran could not answer him; this was a question for those higher than he. White knew that, of course. But the world was changing, and he was an impatient man. "How long will we have to wait before theologians catch up with us?" he asked.[29] The warning turned out to be prescient.

It hadn't been backward technology that kept surgeons from performing beating-heart transplants; it had been the fear of being first. Once Barnard had set the precedent, there would be another 117 heart transplant surgeries in 1968 alone, performed by teams in 18 countries.[30] One of these took place in Virginia—where four doctors would soon stand accused of killing a man in order to take his heart. The deepest anxieties of transplant surgeons like Murray suddenly made national news, as the press conjured images of predatory doctors and "suicide assistance squads,"[31] revealing more starkly than ever that questions of life and death could not be left well enough alone.

## UNLAWFUL HARVEST

On May 25, 1968, Bruce Tucker, a fifty-four-year-old Black man, fell off a concrete wall at the egg-packing plant where he worked.[32] He suffered massive brain damage—a subdural hematoma and brain stem contusion—and slipped into a coma. Two chief physicians at the Medical College of Virginia, Dr. Richard Lower and Dr. David Hume, claimed that "recovery [was] nil and death imminent."[33] Hume and Lower were transplant surgeons.

Tucker's EEG flatlined shortly after he arrived at the hospital; at 3:30 that afternoon, Dr. Lower recommended the respirator be turned off; at 3:35, he pronounced Tucker dead. Less than an hour later, surgeons had removed both his kidneys and cut open his chest—and by the end of the day, Tucker's heart was beating in the body of Joseph Klett, a retired (white) executive.

Hume and Lower were already considered problematic figures for making too-hasty decisions. Hume had himself only recently been acquitted in a wrongful death case for taking the organs of a beating-heart donor; now he had violated Virginia law by declaring Tucker among the "unclaimed dead" almost immediately upon the man's arrival at the hospital, rather than waiting the proper twenty-four hours for his family to be notified.[34] After all, the family might not have agreed to let the hospital use Tucker's organs, and the surgeons didn't want to wait—especially not after determining him a match for Klett. Tucker's brother, William, sued the surgeons who performed the transplant, as well as MCV and others, for wrongful death—but not on the grounds that the surgeons had ignored the requisite waiting period, or even that socioeconomic and racial biases were at work.[35] Instead, he argued that his brother had *still been alive* when his organs were cut out—that it was the transplant surgeons who had killed him.[36] With the removal of Bruce Tucker's beating heart, the problem of brain death left the realm of conjecture and entered the American courtroom.

The racial implications of the Tucker case gave the lawsuit special relevance in 1968 America. Martin Luther King Jr. had been assassinated in Memphis that March, and it was no accident that William Tucker chose a civil rights lawyer, Douglas Wilder (soon to be the first Black man elected to the Virginia Senate the following year), to fight the physicians in court. When the Tucker case hit the presses, the *Baltimore Afro-American* argued that "medical researchers were preparing Black people to be spare parts for whites," and an article titled "Heart Taken, Not Given" ran in major papers including the *Boston Globe*, the *Los Angeles Times*, and the *Washington Post*.[37] The lawsuit dredged up memories of injustices from the previous century, when doctors could not procure medical specimens legally and so occasionally resorted to stealing from newly dug graves. The bodies of Black people and the poor were principal targets; some never even made it from the hospital to the burial ground before ending up on dissection tables. Body donation programs and strict laws had put an end to the practice, but now its ghost had risen again. Even the location of Tucker's death—in Virginia, at a hospital with an already tense relationship with the local Black community—added to suspicions that race had factored into the decision to remove Tucker from life support. This was a state whose law against interracial marriage had only just been repealed.[38]

The concept of brain death did not sit easy with most people, but the suggestion of a new traffic in bodies stung with the poison of slavery and the ongoing fight for civil rights. The *Philadelphia Tribune* even speculated that while "Black medical experts shied away from using the word 'genocide,' the not too distant example of the Jews in Nazi Germany who were used in 'medical experiments' . . . obviously was on their minds."[39] Others perhaps thought of the Russian gulag, where experiments recorded on grainy black-and-white film revealed living men strapped down so their brains might be poked at through openings drilled into their skulls.

The fear wasn't merely that new technology was ripe for abuse. In Cleveland, the *Call & Post*, a historically Black newspaper, questioned the entire enterprise of transplants. After all, Mr. Klett, the recipient of Bruce Tucker's heart, had died not long after his "lifesaving" surgery. Nearly fifteen years after the first kidney transplant, less than 25 percent of transplant recipients lived for more than a year.[40] Even though the odds were improving, it seemed like a lot of resources (not to mention ethical quandaries) for only modest success. "There is something unnatural" about twentieth-century man, the *Call & Post* editorial proclaimed. Every day he worked to solve problems in science, but didn't seem to care about social problems like racism and civil rights. No, the surgeon himself risked becoming "void of emotions, ruthless, cruel, an empty shell not an image of any kind of God, but an image of nothingness."[41] As the race riots that began in the aftermath of Martin Luther King's assassination in April 1968 continued around the nation that summer, readers in Cleveland must have wondered if the editorial board was right.

By 1968 Cleveland's Black community, almost as old as the city itself, made up almost 40 percent of the city's population.[42] Many members had been forced into east-side ghettos as the gap widened between the (white) haves and (Black) have-nots. On July 23, 1968, shots rang out in the city's Glenville neighborhood, sparking several days of riots that resulted in the National Guard's interference. Three policemen were killed in the conflict, and Louis Stokes, Cleveland's first Black mayor, found himself pulling all white police officers from the neighborhood.[43] Though Fred Evans, a Black nationalist leader, would ultimately be held accountable for inciting the events, it was only too clear that the Glenville riots had their roots in segregation, poverty, and racism.[44] Those problems would have been painfully apparent at Cleveland Metropolitan General Hospital, which had been one of the first hospitals in town to desegregate. It still saw the greatest contingent of the city's urban poor, and so a larger proportion of its impoverished minorities. The *Call & Post* editorial didn't mention any surgeons at Metro by name, although it's likely the article would have reached some of White's multiracial staff. Whether they thought it an accurate description of White, we can't know.

In White's interview with Father Curran three months before the riots broke out, the surgeon had made a single mention of the rising tensions at home. "If I were perfectly honest with myself," he admitted as the interview wound down, "I'd forget all this scientific research jazz and go down to the ghettos of Cleveland" to treat poor patients for free.[45] But White didn't leave the research lab, and while he hired one of the most diverse groups of technicians and surgeons in any department at Metro—his medical staff was composed of white, Black, Hispanic, and Asian members, though all from similar socioeconomic backgrounds—he never engaged directly with issues of race and transplant. White had progressive ideas for the 1960s, but much as the *Call & Post* editorial observed, he never considered the solving of racial injustice to be the province of medicine.

The *Call & Post* wasn't the only periodical to become disillusioned with the medical establishment. The media that had once proclaimed Christiaan Barnard's heart transplant a miracle would change its tune within a year. Albert Rosenfeld, a writer for *Life* magazine, demanded a moratorium on heart transplants, and at least one biologist called for Barnard himself to be disbarred.[46] The *New York Times* published an editorial that mirrored the *Baltimore Afro-American*'s language, noting the threat transplant posed to all Americans. "Can anyone ever again be sure that doctors will do all that can be done to save him—rather than regard him as a potential spare-parts supermarket for the propping up of someone else?" the paper asked.[47] Barnard responded by calling an international meeting in Cape Town, where he publicly denounced those he saw as inhibiting progress. "If you have a patient who can fulfill the criteria for becoming a potential donor once you stop the respirator, you can also be certain that the patient will die," he insisted, "so why wait until the heart stops beating?"[48]

The reason, of course, was that to many, the heart is more than a mere pump, and emotional attachment was far stronger than science had anticipated.[49] That four-chambered muscle, constricting in darkness but always reassuring in its steady thrumming beat, awoke concerns that kidney transplants had not. Fears surfaced about what technology could next achieve. Where would it end? Who had the authority to decide? Three months into 1968, White had warned Father Curran that theologians would find themselves painted into a corner, should science be allowed to move ahead without the ethical engagement of religious leaders. Two years later, White would make good on that claim by bringing the argument for brain death all the way to Rome.

## MR. HUMBLE MEETS THE POPE

The pope does not make house calls. Usually. Instead, visitors gather at a special entrance off Saint Peter's Square in Vatican City, where they are met by Pontifical Swiss Guards, resplendent in multicolored robes as bright as harlequin jesters. From there, the public is ushered into a grand audience room.[50] Elbows squeeze elbows from one jammed pew to the next, and when the pope enters, wild applause erupts. American Catholics, even the most enthusiastic of celebrants, can scarcely conceive of the pulsating energy; one of White's friends (a former Cleveland mayor) described it as roaring and carousing as Cleveland's West Side Market on a Saturday.[51] As a general audience member, White would have been at the epicenter of dancing pilgrims, music, and singing, the Swiss Guards' regalia blending into the costumes worn by travelers from all over the world.

But White would not be among the general audience.

For years, White had referred to himself as "Humble Bob." His colleagues winced at the nickname. It was a joke, mostly: *There is nothing humble about Robert White*. White would agree, at least as far as the limelight went; he enjoyed the attention, and expected (and demanded) respect from others in his profession. After the monkey head transplant, he'd enjoyed a suddenly public fame. Already stopped and greeted on the streets of Cleveland—goodwill from his lifesaving surgeries on locals—he'd become known in far corners of the world; Fallaci's article had been translated and reprinted in Italian and Spanish, while German and Russian magazines carried more congenial accounts of the same surgical achievement. International conferences courted his attention, from the International Congress of Neurological Surgery in Tokyo to meetings in Karolinska, London, and Mexico City, along with radio and news programs looking for a quote on brain death and the end of life. There was even a popular joke among the family that should White ever meet the pope, people would ask, "Who is that man with Bob?" Now he stood in the very shadow of the Vatican, the religious center of his world . . . and he hadn't been invited as a supplicant. He'd come to teach.

Vatican City in unexpected sunshine: White wandered the splendid marble courtyard of the Pontifical Academy of Sciences, blistering white under the bright blue sky. Since at least 1936, the academy had investigated scientific subjects through interdisciplinary cooperation, acting as an independent body of the Holy See, with the freedom to research topics without specifically religious overtones. Past academy members from the scientific community, most of them secular, included Nobel Prize winners like Alexis Carrel, whose troubling work transplanting dogs' legs had served as a kind of progenitor of White's own. White had been invited by Jesuit scholars to provide a two-day seminar and a chance to explain his view that brain death equaled human death.[52] They'd asked him personally, *Dr. Robert White*, not Joseph Murray or Henry Beecher or any other member of the Harvard ad hoc committee. He would tell them that the brain held the soul. He'd tell them the problems facing transplantation, problems caused by an alarmist media—and by a Catholic collective reticent to weigh in. But if White was a roaring lion among surgeons, he was still just another lamb in the flock of the Church. He could only preach and hope the Jesuits came around to his way of thinking.

A priest in a simple black cassock waited for White at the end of his last lesson. He approached White, smiling kindly, but he wasn't one of the scholars or students. Would White be available for a brief audience with the Holy Father? the priest asked. The pope, who had been unable to make it to the seminar, nevertheless wanted to inquire about brain death. He wanted White to explain it personally.

Some Catholics wait their entire lives for a glimpse of the pontiff. White now walked on numb feet to meet the man himself. He would describe the elation in later interviews, still breathless with the excitement of it: "Next thing I know, I'm sitting down with Paul VI!"[53] It's a peculiar chance for anyone; it was the chance of a lifetime for Robert White, to be brought into private audience with the pope. Paul VI had a surprising grasp of the issues at hand; he had even spoken to the academy a few years earlier about the spiritual implications of the brain. "Who does not see the close connection between the cerebral mechanism, as they appear from the results of experimentation, and the higher processes which concern the spiritual activity of the soul?" he had asked at the time.[54] This did not amount to an agreement that brain and soul were the same, however. The pope spoke mostly Italian; through an interpreter, White did his best to relate what he'd been saying since well before the present contest over transplants: if a patient was never going to wake up, then he should be determined to be dead even if his body still had a heartbeat.[55] Machines breathing into the tubes of the body, expanding its lungs, causing the basic human engineering to pump and constrict, were merely acting on biological matter. This was no longer a someone, but a something.

Paul VI understood what was at stake; decisions about when life began and ended would have far-reaching implications. He also agreed with White that the Catholic Church should offer its "light" to researchers approaching "the threshold of those grave questions which transcend the domain of science."[56] But he did not give White what he'd most hoped for: there would be no papal decision about the moment of death—no blessing upon the concept of brain death, or upon the practice of harvesting organs from a body with a beating heart. The pope returned the problem of defining death to the doctors, and so removed the Church from potential controversy.[57] White thanked the pope for his words of encouragement, but he packed his bags for home with a frustrating sense of disappointment. If the pope—leader of the Christian world, in White's eyes—had clarified that yes, brain death is really death, it would have lent moral and ethical support to transplant scientists. And Pope Paul VI had considerable political influence; his words reached any country that supported a Catholic diocese—but he was also the only pope ever to address the United Nations (in a speech demanding peace during the Cold War). Like any scientist, White's work depending on funding—and funding, for better or worse, could be swayed by public opinion. Instead, the burden of proof about brain death returned to White and his colleagues. "It's sort of like he put the monkey back on the doctor's back," he complained.[58] He meant it rather literally.

In the year following his return from the Vatican, White performed four more monkey transplants. The creatures lived between six and thirty-six hours on their newly stitched bodies. Surgical complications (failing blood pressure among them) usually ended the primate's life, though the body's rejection of the head would have occurred eventually. After each had come to its end, White anatomized the brains, carving them in slices and looking for any possible abnormality. To all appearances, however, these were *normal* brains; the tissue remained healthy despite its unusual post-body experience.[59] White even adjusted his technique and left more of the brain stem, the part of the "reptile brain" that controlled breathing, meaning the monkey didn't need a respirator. This was, however, as far as he could go. The last successful monkey transplant lived for nine days, breathing on its own and being fed crushed grapes and bits of ice, before succumbing to immune rejection.[60] Immunosuppressants could help preserve the monkeys in their postoperative state for much longer, but it would do no good to try—not when clinical usage for the procedure seemed slow to materialize. Which is to say, not until White had assurances that he could do this on humans in an operating room.

The euphoria of that first successful head transplant hadn't worn off so much as mellowed into a mission. White had not been able to convince the pope to support that mission, at least not yet, but to proceed with something so groundbreaking would require public support. Grant funds to support the study of primate brains was one thing; funding to support clinical application of a surgery that challenged our very conceptions of life, death, mind, and body was quite another. He had to demonstrate beyond a doubt that his work with monkeys could be practically adapted to prolong human lives. White's use of primates to prove the brain could survive deep cerebral hypothermia and prolonged ischemia (restriction of blood supply) was already being trialed in clinical brain surgery.[61] His proof that hypothermic perfusion could preserve a monkey's brain function during circulatory arrest, thus preventing brain damage during massive heart attacks, would soon be standard procedure.[62] He just needed to demonstrate the same for the cephalic transplant.

White would soon be going back to Italy for an international organ transplant conference. He had his eye on a Tokyo conference, too, but his next invitation would have nothing to do with international acclaim. It came as a seemingly innocuous letter from a woman named Catherine Roberts, a geneticist turned animal rights activist, and it would return White to the problem of ethics . . . and race. He could have ignored the invitation, but here was a chance to take his work to the public in a more direct way; Roberts wanted to debate White in the pages of *The American Scholar*, a publication that brought arts, sciences, politics, and public affairs to a wide general audience. This would be his first chance to answer criticism of his ethics directly, something he never had a chance to do with Oriana Fallaci. Her article had put White on the radar of activists like Roberts, but didn't allow for rebuttal. How he fared here would provide a litmus test for the power of animal activism, and just what sort of challenge it might pose to White's ability to win over a public already nervous about the limits (and hubris) of scientific experimentation.

## DR. BUTCHER ENTERS THE DEBATE

A geneticist and microbiologist (and native Californian), Dr. Roberts had recently published a book titled *The Scientific Conscience*, a collection of essays linked by a common theme: their critique of modern science as dehumanizing. Two chapters addressed animal experimentation, which she found unjustifiable; she wanted to debate White on the topic. She had chosen White for a number of reasons, which she laid out in her opening remarks. (Their "debate" in *The American Scholar* would consist of a series of letters to one another, spread out across several issues of the magazine.) For one, she claimed White didn't believe the human brain *could* be transplanted, but carried on with his gruesome, pointless monkey experiments anyway "in the conviction that his studies represent inevitable biological achievements."[63] But Roberts also chose White because on some level, she considered him a hypocrite. Whatever he claimed about his faith or his ethics, she believed he was practicing without a "spiritually enlightened conscience."[64] His work was immoral, he could not distinguish between good and evil, and "whatever his final authority for his choices," she concluded, "it cannot have been Christianity."[65]

This she wrote to Robert J. White, who had only just returned from Rome and his audience with the pope himself. Roberts had only just begun, however. She was, after all, not merely a journalist; she had scientific training, and she made her argument against animal experimentation in both moral and evolutionary terms. First, she explained, the evolution of man has granted him a correspondingly larger understanding of what's morally right; second, the rapid evolution of technology has meant that ethical choices must be made faster and faster. "Are we to become unfeeling robots?" she asked—echoing the Cleveland *Call & Post* in its ambivalence toward futurism. When humans, now largely irreligious, are faced with moral choices, they erroneously looked toward science and scientists to provide authority and answers. The result "is a morally chaotic world that is becoming an almost unbearable place in which to live and die."[66]

Scientists in this brave new world had "increasing power over life and death" and, she argued, an increasing stake in their findings, as research guaranteed their funding and consequently their salaries.[67] This amounted to a conflict of interest. As proof, Roberts turned to transplant surgery and the battles being waged over patients' rights. Physicians, she claimed, were "snatching" organs, hastening the death of some patients in order to save others they considered more worthy of life.[68] Roberts saw herself as an antivivisectionist, as animal rights activists were called in those days, because they were against vivisection, the cutting up of animals for science. She also considered the antivivisection movement a leader in the fight against a morally blind biomedical community. In their desire to rescue the laboratory animal, Roberts claimed that animal rights activists had become the greatest advocates for universally applied ethics. Her argument elided, if not equated, supporting the equal rights of animals considered "lower" than humans to supporting minorities and—by natural extension—the rights of all, human and otherwise.[69]

There was extensive historical precedent here. Philosopher Jeremy Bentham had written as early as 1789 (on the subject of slave plantations) that "blackness of the skin is no reason why a human should be abandoned without redress to [his] tormentor." He went on to muse that the day may come when animals would be given the same rights as humans, based not on whether they spoke or reasoned, but whether they *suffered*.[70] Bentham's words would be recycled in the 1970s by members of the antivivisection movement, particularly by philosopher Peter Singer, who made a comparison between the Black Liberation Movement and what he saw as the urgent need to extend civil rights to animals as well. "The racist violates the principle of equality," Singer argued, and the experimenter does likewise.[71] He named this anti-animal bias *speciesism*.

Roberts didn't use Singer's exact terminology, but she did hold White in contempt for his treatment of vulnerable and "innocent life." Not only did she disagree with White, she emphasized that his work on animals threatened humanity's humanity: "The scores of remnants of mutilated creatures that White has kept alive in the laboratory have made the world a worse place for all of us to live in."[72]

White received Roberts's essay prior to its appearance in print, as agreed, so he could compose his response. Possibly he'd saved it for his evening hours in his study, with classical music playing in the background, long after his wife and children had gone to sleep. Cleveland spring had given way reluctantly to early summer; the empty lot next door had dried enough to serve as a baseball diamond again, and in a month he'd be taking his children to their customary vacation spot on the lake. Bobby was fifteen already, soon to be driving, and Chris was not far behind—baby Ruth had been walking awhile now, and would soon be out of diapers. Sitting down to the work, White may have expected that Roberts would attack his work the way Fallaci had, writing poignantly about monkeys' childlike hands and innocent souls. He would not have been expecting an attack on his faith, nor could he have anticipated that the animal rights activist would link race and organ harvesting. But White would not be outdone, not in print; his answer would be calculated to surprise.

Surrounding him on the study shelves and piled on the floor were those familiar stacks of books. Not just science, but science fiction, too—and literature, the classics. He dusted off a few favorites from Greek mythology, and chose to call his response "Antivivisection: The Reluctant Hydra." Many-headed and serpentine, the Hydra lived in Lake Lerna near the city of Árgos. Fearsome enough already, the Hydra's secret weapon came from its ability to regenerate; if you cut off one of its many heads, two more would grow in its place. Antivivisection, White would claim, was just such a monster: science had proven again and again that "the alleviation of human suffering justifies the sacrifice of lower animals," yet every time an attack against animal experiment was stopped in one quarter, it cropped up elsewhere twice as vicious.[73]

To Robert White, those who wanted to end all animal testing were no different than people who feared vaccines and so opened the door to new epidemics based on pathos and skewed evidence. They propagated their kind in the same way, too, preying on the uninformed to create acolytes who would support and expand their causes. We are in danger, White continued, of losing our hard-won gains in disease prevention and surgical innovation. Lobby groups had already tried to influence

electorates, attempting to get Congress to restrict the freedom of scientists to pursue research. "The public is tragically unaware," White
wrote, "that progress in medical science is continually threatened by the
antivivisection movement."[74] Because federal research grants provided
the means of vital progress in medicine, laws restricting animal research would affect the health and well-being of the "entire citizenry."[75]
White's "proprietary interest," he wrote with surprising honesty, was the
continued use of animals in experiment. That, he claimed, was all Roberts had any ground to debate with him, and he would neither hear nor
respond to any other attack.

The life of a monkey or the life of a human child? White lay the
choices before the reader with excoriating detail. "Just yesterday," he
wrote, "I removed a tumor from the cerebellum and brain stem of a
small child."[76] The malignancy had been growing, greedily gobbling
up room and increasing pressure inside the brain. The infant suffered
wretched, eye-piercing headaches and continual vomiting. Soon he
could not walk, use his hands, or see. All he knew was pain and discomfort, with no understanding of why it was happening, and no means of
comfort while his helpless parents looked on. Without intervention,
the child was sure to suffer a horribly painful death, but White took
out the tumor without any damage to the child's brain. "That surgery
would have been impossible a few decades ago," White wrote—yet now,
it was routine, and all because of experiments he'd originally performed
on animals.[77] What would the antivivisectionist prefer? he asked. That
we let children die? That we experiment on human beings? Because
(and here he quotes the eminent early twentieth-century brain surgeon
Harvey Cushing) "those who oppose the employment of animals . . .
leave us the only alternative of subjecting our fellow man . . . to our first
crude manipulations."[78]

Activists had been agitating him since Fallaci's article about

"Libby" in 1968, sometimes through published op-eds, occasionally by sending angry letters to the hospital. The more aggressive organizations, White complained, had installed him as their "*célèbre terrible*," their monster scientist, perpetrator of abominable crimes.[79] He followed this declaration by saying that if they wished to accuse him, then he joined the "distinguished company" of men like Drs. Louis Pasteur and Joseph Lister (who brought us into the age of germ theory), Sir Victor Horsley (the first surgeon to remove a brain tumor), and Alfred Blalock (a pioneer in the treatment of shock)—all of whom also experimented on animals. In fact, he wrote, if the use of animals must be abolished, then antivivisectionists must be willing to also live without open-heart surgery, antiseptic, insulin, vaccines, and almost every other breakthrough medicine had derived. These, too, were based upon animal models. Experiments on the monkey brain had allowed White "to unlock many of the subtle mysteries surrounding cerebral function" and so helped create therapies for neurological disease.[80] But like the scientists in Michael Crichton's then-recent bestseller *The Andromeda Strain*, while they worked to save lives in laboratory isolation, public attention outside that protected space had been growing ugly against them. Animal rights activists had successfully manipulated an uninformed public into seeing enemies where none existed. If "allied biological professions" didn't unite to undo the damage, White concluded in his first essay, then the entire nation would suffer.[81]

The debate continued over two further responses between the pair—and characteristically, White got the last word. "I've realized after careful consideration," he wrote in his final essay, penned on his way to Russia for an international transplant conference, that this had all been just a stunt "to amplify [Roberts's] personal religious views"— by which he meant the antivivisection movement. Roberts failed to distinguish one life from another, and in equating "the vegetable and the animal . . . [and] the man," it was Roberts, not White, who lacked humanity.[82]

Life—human life—superseded all else for White, even suffering. He had proof of the moral rightness of this viewpoint, too. The injured soccer player he'd treated two years previous had recently returned to Metro, and so had the young resident who'd once suggested he might be better off dead. The young doctor had been away on rotation for a few years; when he saw the soccer player's name, he was horrified: "Has he been here this whole time?" White only smiled and ushered him into a room where a young and attractive woman waited; this, White explained, was the patient's wife. The now tetraplegic man was only there for a kidney stone; in the interim years, he had fallen in love and married. He and his wife lived together in Romania. They were planning to have children. The resident doctor stared in joyful, awe-struck amazement. White wasn't just teaching medicine; the lesson he meant his doctors and nurses to learn had to do with the uniqueness of the human spirit—and with the sanctity of human life.[83] How could Roberts, or anyone from the antivivisection movement, dare claim the moral high ground over him?

In the end, the *American Scholar* exchange didn't have the reach or the international flair of Fallaci's *Look* article, and promised to do little to change minds on either side. White likely considered the debate a footnote, forgettable and dismissed. He'd certainly dismissed Catherine Roberts. White had other matters to turn his attention to, including the rapidly concluding lawsuit brought by Bruce Tucker's family against the surgeons in Virginia. He couldn't know then that his clash with animal rights had only begun.

Richmond, Virginia, May 18, 1972: The jurors and plaintiffs filed into the city's Law and Equity Court. The doctors who had taken Bruce

Tucker's heart had waited four years for the case to come to trial at last, and now surgeons across the country were paying very close attention.

The suit, for $100,000 in damages, would be focused upon the crucial question as yet unanswered by religion or science: When does death occur? In his opening statement, Douglas Wilder, the Tucker family's lawyer, charged the surgeons with prepping Klett for surgery as soon as Bruce Tucker was admitted, *before* declaring Tucker deceased. "If they had waited even another twenty-four hours," Wilder claimed, "he might have started to recover."[84] While this was not very likely (the injury Tucker sustained had been massive and probably would have led to permanent coma), no one could prove otherwise, and due to the surgeons' actions, we can *never* know. The jury was aghast, and papers reported that prospects for the defense looked grim. After the fourth day, however, Hume and Lower's defense team called their most important medical witnesses: members of the Harvard ad hoc committee. Before the start of the trial, Judge Jude Compton had been deeply suspicious of "brain death," and told the press that he would advise the jurors to "adopt the legal concept of death," not a "medical" one foisted on him by surgeons.[84] But that was about to change.

The case continued for seven days of testimony, but everything came down to the judge's final instructions to the jury on the morning of May 25. Under the law, he explained, death must "occur at a precise time." In order to determine that precise time, the men and women of the jury were permitted to "consider . . . the time of complete and irreversible loss of all function of the brain"—something they could only understand by considering the expertise of the Harvard ad hoc committee, but which would also go *beyond* the committee's report.[86] The committee members had only testified to the definition of permanent coma and the likelihood of death resulting from such a state. The jury would be using that medical expertise to provide an exact moment of death from a legal perspective. Compton admitted that he'd been swayed in recent days by the "consensus of surgeons." The following morning, headlines all across America announced a victory for Lower and Hume: "Virginia Jury Rules that Death Occurs When Brain Dies."[87] In agreeing that death occurs when neurological function ceased in the brain (demonstrated by a flat EEG, among other criteria), they exonerated the physicians from any charges that they caused Tucker's death by removing his still-functioning organs.

After the trial, Dr. Hume said confidently that the court's decision "brings the law up to date with what medicine has known all along—that the only death is brain death."[88] But there was very little that medicine had known "all along." All the careful language in the world cannot paper over the troubling fact that nearly fifty years on, there is still no *medical* definition of death—only a *legal* one. The question is no longer "Are you truly, medically dead when no more brain waves can be detected?" By law, *you are dead enough.*

Whatever White might have felt about the pope's abdication of responsibility for determining the details of when life ends, his own words to Father Curran had been prescient. The decision did, in the end, depend very much on the medical community. Two weeks after the trial ended, an article in the *New York Times* credited Henry Beecher, Joseph Murray, and colleagues with bringing about a revolution in medicine. "Legal acceptance of brain death," the journalist explained, "bolsters the position of transplant teams" and made it easier to take a person off life support, saving the "expense and agony of persisting in a fight for life that has already been lost."[89] Four years earlier, Beecher had cautioned his colleagues on the ad hoc committee to define brain death with the dying patient always foremost in mind—and yet the surgeons had gotten exactly the definition they'd wanted in the end. If a brain-dead body could be treated in the same way as a dead body—its organs removed, care withdrawn—then under American law, life resided in the brain. Just as White had always insisted.

It was a sunny Thursday afternoon, July 6, 1972. The International Transplant Society was gathered in Fiuggi, Italy, for their fifth annual conference. Among the attendees were several Americans, including heart transplant pioneers Michael DeBakey of Houston and Eugene Dong of Palo Alto . . . and a charismatic brain surgeon from Cleveland, Ohio. They did not see many neuroscientists at these meetings. A year earlier, Robert White had attended the First Conference of Neurosurgeons in the USSR, where he'd agreed to an interview on "transplant problems." Asked about his goals for the next decade, he described the "thrilling field of research brain modeling"—of using his isolations as a means of controlling blood flow, cooling the brain, and extending the time available to the brain surgeon for delicate operations.[90] Now, a year later and several months after the first legal decision on brain death, White stood before his colleagues with a different message. "Transplanting the brain, which until yesterday was the last frontier, has today been overcome," he announced.[91] "Although not all the problems have been resolved, today we must, we want, to think of a head transplant."[92]

White would travel to Japan; he would become a near celebrity in Germany. The headlines buzzed like modern clickbait: "Monkey Lives 36 Hours After Receiving Head Transplant"; "Cleveland Surgeon Tells of 8 Head Transplants"; "Monkeys Help Doctor Get 'Ahead.'"* A little closer to home, in an interview for the *Akron Beacon Journal*, White returned to his favorite metaphor: that of human brains as the final frontier. "I like to think of the brain as inner space," he explained, "just as complex as outer space and as difficult to explore."[93] We support and

---

*From the *Arizona Republic*, *Indianapolis Star*, and *Washington Post*, respectively.

praise the outer-space astronaut, but the man who interferes with the brain—he has trespassed too far. "Ever since we got off from viewing the heart as the center [of the self]," White continued, all of our once-fearful reluctance to operate, isolate, or transplant moved from heart to head. Critics called head transplants "Frankensteinian." They called Dr. White the new Modern Prometheus.[94] *Let them.* White shrugged off the epithet more easily than any other. Because his critics didn't understand Frankenstein the way he did.

"It is true that medical science now believes that the definition of death is an integral part of brain function, so that when the brain is dead, then the patient, the person is dead," White said in 1972, appearing for the first time on grainy televisions through a local Ohio station.[95] "The literature has run ahead of us in terms of brain transplantation. [Because head transplant] in a sense, has already been solved"—not by medicine, but by Mary Shelley, by Victor Frankenstein.[96] White wanted to extend life, to let his patients live better lives, and longer ones. He saw Frankenstein's quest as the same, though warped by the desire to create a new creature rather than preserving the life of God's own. To be called a Modern Prometheus, to be considered in the same realm of gods breathing new life into men, bringing light into darkness and leading the way to a future where possibility outstripped desire—this was no disparagement. "We venture into the void," White said with the same bright quickening of first love. "The maps and pathways of the brain are less well-marked and more subtle than those taken by astronauts."[97] Breaking boundaries wasn't an accident along the way; it was the whole enterprise. This is the path, he announced during that 1972 Italian symposium, "and we will go on."[98]

# Chapter 7

# THE HUMAN ANIMAL

"*The camera adds ten pounds, Robert.*"

White would be making several appearances on Cleveland's late-night *Big Chuck and Lil' John Show*, adding some local color to comedy skits attacking Pittsburgh Steelers fans (the number one rivals of the Cleveland Browns). "Is this beneath my dignity?" he'd asked Patricia, who had raised an eyebrow. "Don't be a fuddy-duddy," she told him.[1] It wasn't that White had any real reticence about appealing to pop culture; a preeminent surgeon's public engagement, he believed, was an honor and a duty, and his fellow scientists just weren't very good at it. But the nagging worry about his personal presentation wouldn't go away. White's broad and stocky frame had always provided ample undercarriage for extra weight. In his mid-fifties and now entirely bald, his round face and round middle cut what he considered an unflattering figure for stage and screen. Deciding something must be done, White started skipping breakfasts. Then he skipped lunches, too. Eventually, the surgeon's weight loss plan consisted of coffee, Diet Coke, and a trough of salad at dinner. A terrible health plan, to be sure, but White was finding himself increasingly in the public eye—and that wasn't likely to change.

The fight over brain death had proved that even research scientists ignored public opinion at their peril. American progress in heart transplant medicine had stalled while the lawsuit disputing science's claim to Bruce Tucker's heart had wound its way through the courts. As soon as twelve Virginian jurors affirmed the surgeons' right to harvest organs from the brain-dead man, transplant cases rose quickly. Experts could continue to debate the exact definition of death, but for most people, the *New York Times* headlines in the weeks after the trial offered a simpler truth: brain death equaled real death. Money for experiments from big, taxpayer-funded entities like the National Institutes of Health swiftly followed, but competition to get those funds greatly increased, too. The systems that undergirded science relied more on public opinion than most were willing to admit. And now that the public had accepted the good that came from transplanting the heart, why not the brain?

White had been so sure the time was coming—*People* magazine had called his work "revolutionary," had hailed his monkey brain isolations and transplants as among the key discoveries in a quarter century.[2] Still, he understood that there were those among the public who remained intent on seeing such work as unethical, morbid, *wrong*. And so White embarked on something of a world tour to educate the masses, if he could, about what he called "the rights and wrongs of fabricated man."[3] (Those who attend his lectures would learn there were, in fact, no wrongs—not in White's mind, anyway. The only wrong was to deny surgeons the chance to experiment.) He'd spent years going to conferences at home and abroad, trying to convince his colleagues that his was not "fringe" science. But when White turned to the public, he chose a different tack. Instead of arguing that his work was *not*

Frankensteinesque, he defended Victor Frankenstein as a pioneer, writing as much in popular magazines such as *Reader's Digest* and *People*. He even appeared at a benefit ball at Halloween dressed in a Victorian topcoat with *Dr. Frankenstein* emblazoned on his medical bag. For good or ill, White knew how to make headlines.

Several of White's children had gone off to college now, and every Sunday, he used a ruler to make a new chore grid for the remaining kids at home—a bit of long-distance parenting for the weeks he spent away. He made regular calls to Shaker Heights and wrote sometimes, too; "Dearest Patty," he wrote from Paris, "set down to writing you a real letter!" complete with a heart beneath the exclamation point.[4] He promised to take her with him on the next trip to Russia, asked after the classes she'd been taking at the university, how she was managing to write term papers in the middle of the night when the kids finally conked out.

But as White endeavored to convince an international public that transplanting a brain was no less ethical than transplanting a kidney or a heart, he began to realize that he was engaged in the wrong debate. His audiences had developed other, more pressing concerns—not about the morality of playing around with the soul, but about the morality of even the most basic biological research involving animals. In 1980, some members of the animal rights community (which included different schools of thought) had joined together to establish People for the Ethical Treatment of Animals (PETA), an organization through which they could lobby for laws that would limit research facilities' ability to purchase animals from the pound, allow humans to file suits on behalf of animals, and introduce new regulations for animals' rights to a better life. Through the work of its founders, especially Ingrid Newkirk, PETA grabbed the public's attention—even hosting its own televised rock concerts on MTV. By the decade's end, White's flair for public confrontation would make him one among their rivals—and funding, already elusive, would become tied to whether White satisfied the American public's new passion for animal rights. To continue his research on monkeys—to perfect the techniques he hoped to one day use to transplant the human brain—he would have to face PETA in the court of public opinion.

## SEVENTEEN MONKEYS

On September 11, 1981, police surrounded a laboratory in Montgomery County, Maryland, just outside Washington, DC. The Institute for Behavioral Research occupied an unassuming two-story building in Silver. Orders were given, and enforcement officers entered the mostly empty building over a long weekend break, only to be overwhelmed by the odor of urine and feces.[5] As they approached the "colony room," as it was called, the smell became unbearable. Seventeen macaque monkeys from the Philippines peered out of small, dirty cages. Some were missing digits. Others had open sores on their arms and legs.[6] "Gloves on," Lieutenant Richard Swain commanded. It was too unsanitary to work any other way. "I've executed lots and lots of search warrants. I've worked in murder, in narcotics, in vice, but this was the first time I went into a room and I felt legitimately concerned for my health just being there," he later told a reporter from the *Washington Post*.[7] It was the first police raid of a research facility in Maryland—in the whole country, in fact—and it had been made possible by a man named Alex Pacheco, the cofounder of PETA.

"I first discovered animal rights in 1978," Pacheco explained in an article he'd later write about the "Silver Spring 17."[8] A native Ohioan, he'd originally planned to enter the Catholic priesthood, but a visit to a slaughterhouse where a friend worked over summers radically altered his course. Appalled by what he considered the livestock's devastatingly inhumane treatment, he found comfort in the works of Peter Singer.

Singer, a professor of bioethics and a prominent member of the animal rights movement, had written his magnum opus, *Animal Liberation*, just three years before. By 1978, Singer had published a reader with philosopher Tom Regan called *Animal Rights and Human Obligations* that took his ideas further still. While Singer made occasional caveats about experimentation (suggesting that perhaps some was necessary), he and Regan nonetheless argued that the "best" way to use animals for science was simply "not to use them."[9] After the book's publication, a review in the *New York Times* put the number of animals used for experiments yearly at 80 million—a number that included 45 million rats and mice, 700,000 rabbits, 500,000 dogs, and 200,000 cats.[10] Of these, the piece claimed, most contributed "nothing" to biomedical research (in that they did not, in the reviewer's opinion, lead to any fundamental benefits). Not that it mattered what came from the animals' deaths—their sacrifice was a crime in and of itself. "Death is the ultimate harm because it is the ultimate loss," Regan insisted; animals should not be viewed as expendable.[11] Like the human animal, they had feelings, and they deserved equal rights. The young Pacheco readily agreed. He became an eager convert, and two years later in 1980—by then a political science and environmental studies major at George Washington University—he joined forces with a seasoned activist named Ingrid Newkirk.

Born in England, Newkirk had moved to India when young and volunteered alongside her mother aiding Mother Teresa's work on leprosy. Her interest in protecting animals began while she was still abroad, and after moving to the United States, Newkirk spent eleven years working for animal rights as DC's first woman poundmaster. Adept at introducing legislation to support and regulate spay and neuter clinics and provide public funding for veterinary services, Newkirk closely followed the movements of international organizations like the United Kingdom's Animal Liberation Front. She, too, had read Singer's work, and from her own experience with animal welfare she became convinced that the United States needed its own grassroots group for animal liberation. Pacheco would soon seek out Newkirk, and his zeal and energy would prove invaluable to her cause.[12] First, however, they needed to build their reputation, and to do that they needed to choose a name, a focus, and a place to begin. After deciding upon their moniker, People for the Ethical Treatment of Animals, Newkirk and Pacheco determined to focus first on animals used in medical experimentation, which had been the backbone of the nascent antivivisectionist movement at the dawn of the twentieth century.* Pacheco had already done some background research and knew about the Institute for Behavioral Research in Silver Spring; next he would seek to gain personal experience of its practices. He applied to an open position, and in a matter of days was installed as a student volunteer under Dr. Edward Taub, whose remit was to perform experiments on surgically crippled primates to monitor the rehabilitation of impaired limbs.[13]

Taub had been running tests on deafferentation, which involved severing the "dorsal roots" of the spinal nerves, which carry sensory input from the limbs to the central nervous system.[14] In essence, it meant rendering the monkey incapable of *feeling* its limbs, but not paralyzed from *moving* them. He would then stimulate the monkeys in various

---

*Called the "Brown Dog Affair," the controversy that birthed the antivivisection movement in Britain centered on man's best friend and played upon public sympathy for the grim deaths of laboratory dogs.

ways—from promises of food to electric shocks—to make the animal move the deafferented limb. Macabre it was, but the work essentially overturned a mistaken assumption in neuroscience (established in the 1890s, also by severing monkey nerves) that a lack of feeling caused paralysis of a limb. By 1982, Taub's research was in its ninth year of funding—the first seven provided for by the National Institute of Mental Health, and subsequently by the NIH.[15] Taub's thesis was one of "learned non-use": the only reason monkeys didn't use their numb limbs was because they had not "learned' (or relearned) to do so. He held out hope that human beings might ultimately be taught to reuse deafferented body parts, too, and funding agencies agreed. The NIH hoped the research would yield rehabilitation protocols for human stroke victims.[16] Everything was going Taub's way, and when Taub returned home after hiring Pacheco, he bragged to his wife, "What a marvelous student I have. He took the position without any pay, purely out of interest!"[17] He didn't realize just how much interest, or why.

Pacheco left the lab on his first day deeply troubled. The sight of monkeys strapped into a boxlike contraption built from an old refrigerator and then forced to move, sometimes goaded with electric shocks, sickened him. He didn't believe any animal should be made to undergo such treatment, nor did he think the ends (helping stroke victims) justified the means. But going public with his personal offense at these experiments would have no effect on Taub's lab. After all, animal studies were legal and government-funded. Instead, Pacheco focused on the *conditions* the animals found themselves in. "I saw filth caked on the wires of the cages, feces piled in the bottom of the cages, urine and rust encrusting every surface," he wrote in an article that would be published, appropriately, in a new book by Peter Singer. "There, amid this rotting stench, sat sixteen crab-eating macaques and one rhesus monkey, their lives limited to metal boxes just 17 and 3/4 inches wide."[18]

The monkeys had grown neurotic, spinning endlessly in their cages, biting off the fingers they could not feel, and chewing holes in their own limbs. Pacheco showed Newkirk the photos he had secretly taken of an "acute noxious stimuli test," where monkeys were placed in an immobilizing chair and a "stimulus" (such as surgical pliers) attached to their testicles. A monkey named Domitian had been used as the "example." PETA now had a face and a name to distribute to the press. Still, they had to be careful. The evidence needed to do more than move the public; it also had to stand up in court.

Fortunately for Pacheco and Newkirk, Taub had made it all too easy. The scientist had a research trip in August and had already given Pacheco keys to the lab. With full confidence and no prying eyes, Pacheco invited five scientists experienced in primate behavior to witness the laboratory's conditions, bringing them in secretly, one at a time. By then, the lab was at its worst. Taub had only one regular animal technician, a man named John Kunz, and the operation relied on student assistants for cleanup. With the doctor away, the students didn't come in regularly.[19] Pacheco's guests stood aghast at the wretched conditions and sickening smell. They signed five affidavits, each claiming that the cages were caked and filthy and the smell overpowering; four also noted that the monkeys were living in constant harsh light with no restful darkness due to a broken timer. All cited unnecessary animal suffering.[20] Soon after, with their expert testimony in hand, Pacheco and Newkirk convinced local authorities to get a warrant for seizure. The raid took place a few weeks later, resulting in the removal of Taub's primates. The sting marked the beginning of a long legal battle, every bit as important as the one fought over brain death and heart transplant. It unfolded in the public spotlight, and PETA made sure to be front and center.

· · ·

When Lieutenant Swain arrived on the morning of the raid, a gathering of news media flocked noisily around the edges of activity. Pacheco had violated Maryland law, inviting the press for what should have been a classified search and seizure. Incensed, Swain ordered the reporters away, but it was much too late; the "Silver Spring Monkeys" became international news—with Domitian's pitiful portrait as the leading image. The raid would result in two criminal trials; one in 1981 prosecuting Taub for animal cruelty, and a second on appeal in 1982, wherein Taub earned his acquittal. It would also pit the NIH, whose funding had been used for the purchase and care of the monkeys, against Congress in a custody battle over who could take charge of them.*

PETA had discovered the power of lobbying. In their fight for rights to the Silver Spring monkeys, they managed to win over Representative Robert C. Smith, who drafted a petition on their behalf. In the end, 253 House members and 52 senators signed, but still the NIH refused to hand them over, citing a pending court case. PETA followed what would become their protocol and went to the public—and to the streets in protest. *Nature* published stories about the case, calling the monkeys the most celebrated icons of animal rights in the country, and a documentary would be filmed in their honor. Doris Day, who had retired from films to become an avid defender of animals, called the monkeys "political prisoners." Protests swamped the White House and 46,000 letters would be sent to then First Lady Barbara Bush before the custody case made it to the Supreme Court.[21]

Meanwhile, Taub was also taking the stand. The charges against him originally numbered 113, violations that included sharp protruding

---

*Complications over whether state anti-cruelty laws applied to federally funded research muddied matters further.

cage wires, no feed bowls, nothing for healthy cognitive stimulation, lighting problems, fecal matter, and a possible infestation of mice. Two veterinarians, Drs. Ott and Robinson, examined the primates (seven nonsurgical animals and ten that had been surgically altered). Most of the nonsurgical animals were reportedly in good health, though one was undernourished; of the ten others, six had minor treatment needs, two for what appeared to be bone fractures that had healed poorly. The remaining four needed urgent veterinary care to drain lesions and wounds, and all the monkeys had missing or mangled digits.[22]

In the end, Taub would only be found guilty of six counts of cruelty to animals. He admitted that the lab was in poor condition on the day of the raid, but insisted that this was anomalous and due to his vacation, citing prior USDA inspection reports that indicated only minor infractions. He also seemed to suggest that the fault lay with Kunz's "demure nature" (presumably for not forcing the student assistants to clean more regularly) and even with Pacheco, for not contacting him about the mess.[23] Even the scientists brought by Pacheco could not agree that the situation constituted abuse in the strictest sense. In fact, all the testimony had essentially canceled out, with one set of experts calling the lab filthy, and the next calling it reasonably clean. As a result, Taub was held accountable only for failing to provide proper veterinary care to six monkeys, and fined $3,000.

Taub later claimed that details of the lab's condition had been staged, miscommunicated, or fabricated entirely. He called the trial a blow to all science, a witch hunt, and compared his treatment by PETA to being burned at the stake. In speaking of PETA, Taub insisted "we're not dealing with a benign adversary . . . They're extremely dangerous and extremely malicious and they'll do anything. And it is minor to them to destroy a person."[24]

For Taub, having his name defamed, his lab raided, and his grant canceled effectively rendered him without a salary or the means of doing further research. He appealed, however, and won acquittal on five of the six charges, meaning he had only been guilty of one act of negligence to one monkey, which had to have its arm amputated. It would be 1986 before he was permitted to work again, thanks to a grant from the University of Alabama—but despite the years of fighting with PETA, Taub was not ruined. His work on deafferentation ultimately bore fruit. The final examination of the euthanized monkeys (performed through the offices of the NIH) proved that their brains had begun remapping communication to their numb limbs. Taub subsequently developed a new form of therapy, based on the concept of neuroplasticity, for people disabled by stroke. The Society for Neuroscience would cite Taub's work as one of the twentieth century's top ten accomplishments in neuroscience.[25]

In some ways, the most poignant thing to come out of the case wasn't the legal decision, or the consequences for Edward Taub. It's what it meant *publicly*. PETA wasn't just the work of two dedicated activists and their small band of associates; it was the fastest-growing animal rights group in America.[26] As *Washington Post* correspondent Peter Carlson put it, the Silver Spring 17 aided PETA, only a year old, in building a large and aggressive movement not just against cruelty to lab animals, but toward a new relationship between humans and animals.[27] When the NIH tried to get the monkeys back and sent to a different lab, where the work they'd funded could continue, PETA's savvy tactics for media coverage sparked a public outburst of disapproval that brought the project to a halt (again). PETA would never successfully get custody of the monkeys, and ultimately, the NIH would manage to perform a final experiment on three that had been slated to be euthanized due to their poor health. But as a result of PETA's interference, four of the survivors would find homes in the San Diego Zoo.

No other lab would be raided in the way Taub's had been; there would be no need. Pacheco spoke of the success in psychological terms: "It scared the bejesus out of a bunch of experimenters."[28] They wouldn't dare mistreat animals now. The media had helped PETA refocus the public's attention: it was no longer a question of *how* to use experimental animals, but *whether* to use them at all. PETA had power. And, in the eyes of many, they also had the moral upper hand.

## WHAT EXPERIMENTS ARE MADE FOR

Activists and media outlets like the *New York Times* suggested animal experiments had no purpose and achieved no outcomes—or, that the taking of animal life was not worth the knowledge obtained. PETA, using the megaphone of its success, called animal researchers immoral, unethical, brutal. White bristled at such statements. He claimed that every scientific breakthrough, from antiseptic to vaccines, had been earned by dint of effort and practice that would not have been possible without animal test subjects. He could show them the results . . . But these opponents weren't interested in the ends, just the means. You are destroying a life, they said. A life they found as valuable as any human's.

In White's first encounter with the antivivisectionists, his debate with Catherine Roberts (a version of which would be published later in the *New York Times Sunday Magazine*, and included in the 1988 edition of Singer and Regan's book), he had suggested a hierarchy: humans were permitted to benefit at the cost of "lower animals." He supported this claim by describing the human brain, and by inference the human being, as "the most complex and superbly designed structure" known to man.[29] As to considering humans above the other animals, even the primates? "I will not argue it," he stated again and again.[30] However much he might belittle what he called "the theology of the antivivisection movement," what White takes for granted in each essay is that the human has a soul and the animal has none.

As Newkirk and Pacheco arranged their raid on Dr. Taub's Silver Spring lab, White had been busy establishing the Vatican's new biomedical ethics commission. As leader of the committee, White finally had his chance to shape the church's stance on brain death—and on in vitro fertilization, the other side of life's beginning and end. Biomedical ethics were literally his domain, an honor bestowed upon him by the pope himself, as God's representative. And over the years, the Catholic Church's stance on brain death would shift to one more in keeping with White's own. Next to that, the animal rights debate seemed tedious, small. "Animal usage is not a moral or ethical issue and elevating the problem of animal rights to such a plane is a disservice to medical research," White would insist.[31] The death of animals did not please him, but it didn't come close to the feeling he experienced when he lost a patient. A human life, a *child's* life, was infinitely more valuable to him. In surgery, White knew that beneath his cramping fingers pulsed the substrate of a person's highest functions. Personality. Intelligence. Free will. White might give lectures all day about brain death, about *when* a patient died. But he couldn't say *why*. He thought about his own sons and daughters; he thought about the parents; he thought about their hopes and dreams. And White—White *prayed*: "Please, God, give strength to my hands."[32]

Catholic doctrine told him that God's plans weren't man's plans. God didn't explain why people died, like the veteran whose thirteen-year-old daughter would pack away the get-well cards because they could not send his brain cancer into remission.[33] Or the eighteen-year-old girl, hit by a drunk driver, who never regained consciousness, living on life support in a care facility—what White called "a cemetery for living monuments."[34] People died, were paralyzed, were trapped inside their bodies as a living mind with no way out. He wanted to know how to help them; he wanted to know why something worked and why it didn't.[35] And for all that, he needed to map the brain in every complexity, try every surgery, examine branch after branch of every arterial connection. He only understood the mysterious terrain of the human brain because he'd mapped the brains of primates—because, in effect, he had monkeys to practice on.

PETA would claim that primates took priority over the depraved theoretical questions of science. And White's head transplants, the flashiest of his experiments, might be hard to defend against PETA's assault. But White's work saved lives—specific lives, little girls' lives. And *that*, he would insist, was what experiments were made for.

In 1981, shortly after PETA's successful infiltration of Taub's lab, White met with a young patient at Metro. He had known Caroline* since she was quite small; she was always cheerful, with white-blond hair tied back in ribbons. Now eleven years of age, she also wore thick bangs. Her brain's vascular system had developed on the *outside* of her skull, and a bright blue vein was visible through the pale skin of her forehead. When she was standing, it was less noticeable; once seated, it appeared as a branching blue tree—and should she lay her head back, it became blue-purple and hard as a rock; the tissue surrounding it would swell and tense. The slightest cut or bruise to that sensitive place could cost the girl her life.[36] White had never seen this type of malformation before. But nearly all his work on monkeys had to do, in one way or another, with the vascular systems of the cranium. He determined to begin an experimental protocol to try to fix the anomaly. It meant more monkeys; it also meant taking time away from any further research on

---

*Names have been altered to protect the identity of the patient.

transplants—but that was a sacrifice he was willing to make. He was a brain surgeon; transplant was but one area of his expertise. Yes, it was his favorite—one he'd gladly spend his life perfecting. But here, in his hospital, was a patient who needed him *now*. The human soul could wait.

Caroline's brain, nestled inside her skull, had not entirely severed its ties with the outside world. The veins of her scalp remained interconnected with the veins feeding her brain itself, and in her short life, these growing and pulsing vessels had eroded holes right through the bone of the skull.[37] Somehow, White needed to cut through those veins that were on the wrong side; but in destroying them, Caroline could bleed to death or suffer a stroke. He needed to develop a technique that allowed him to close the blood vessels as he severed them. He needed, in addition, to *practice*.

White's team had, since their first brain isolation in 1963, experimented repeatedly with the tying-off and reconnecting of veins and arteries. With the assistance of microneurosurgeon Dr. Yoshiro Takaoka, White had recently performed a "vascular split" of the monkey brain, separating the vessels of the right and left hemispheres using ligatures.[38] His team had simultaneously been perfecting the use of new tools for stemming blood flow from incisions. Reporter Oriana Fallaci had described the smell of burning flesh as White used a cautery blade to singe and seal tissue as he cut. But times had changed. The Brain Research Lab had been experimenting with new high-precision laser scalpels, as well as a technique that "soldered" vessels to close them in a more efficient and less damaging way than older techniques. All these techniques could be brought to bear on Caroline's surgery—but even after a year of perfecting them, White remained unsatisfied.

"My sincerest apologies for constantly getting your hopes up and dashing them," White wrote to Caroline's parents on June 30, 1982.[39]

Caroline had just turned twelve, and still had to wear a protective helmet and sleep propped up with pillows. "It has always been my feeling that we can accomplish this," but he refused to take any shortcuts, White went on.[40] "What I would like all three of you to do is temporarily forget about" the possibility of surgery, he wrote, and enjoy the first blush of summer.[41] He didn't really think they would—not while watching Caroline's playmates join sports teams and go swimming, jumping, skipping, and climbing in ways she never had, and possibly would never be able to. By August, White had told them. Surely by then? White closed the letter with paternal tenderness, writing of "my own personal concern and love for your daughter." His own youngest child was only two years older than Caroline, and was packing for the family's annual beach trip with a dwindling number of siblings. Still, White had ten healthy children. Ten children who had never been under the neurosurgical scalpel, who had spent their childhoods running bases in the vacant lot. He promised to spend the rest of the summer exhausting himself in the effort to find a way forward to surgery. But the summer would go by. And then the year. The animal experiments carried on.

By June 1983, White felt they could wait no longer. He must act, or concede that nothing could be done for Caroline. During his two years of research, he'd discovered that Caroline's malformation appeared with some consistency in medical literature from China and Japan, but nowhere had he discovered a means of treating it, or a protocol for operating.[42] And so White had developed the techniques from scratch.[43] If the surgery succeeded, it would prove everything White had said about the purpose of his work: use the monkey, save the man. Even so, every surgical expert White consulted advised against proceeding.[44]

But on August 2, 1983, White and his team prepped Caroline for surgery. She wore a silvery nightgown embroidered with a flower and clutched a baby doll and a little gray teddy bear. Her parents waited for her in the family waiting room, wearing trails in the carpet with their pacing; everyone assured them Caroline was the *best* little girl (though, now thirteen, she was growing up before their eyes), well-behaved and polite, even as they shaved her head. Meanwhile, in White's operating room, the surgeons had scaled up the perfusion technology, which waited nearby. White prayed they would not need it, hoping to do the surgery without lowering Caroline's body or brain temperature so they might monitor her brain waves at their usual rates, but he wanted every precaution ready. If too much blood loss occurred, rapid cooling of her brain would preserve it from cell death, as a cold brain requires far less blood-borne oxygen. White planned to use a series of laserlike jets to close up the vessels as they worked beneath her scalp in the hopes that blood flow could be controlled. With everything ready, they propped Caroline in a seated position with just a slight tilt, as if she were in a dentist's chair, and waited for the anesthesia to take effect.[45] Maurice Albin gave the sign when she was fully under, and White made the first cut well behind Caroline's ear. Slowly, carefully, he peeled back her scalp.

White expected large veins communicating through bone to the brain. But he did not find them. Instead, there were dozens and dozens of very small vessels connecting the scalp and cranial circulation. "We won't need the perfusion," White said with obvious relief. Instead, they began individually destroying each of the small connecting vessels with the jetlike cautery, obliterating the tiny skull holes with wax. "Closing the wound," White announced, and they sewed careful stitches along the top of Caroline's shaved head and applied a tight dressing of bandages. It had gone remarkably smoothly—the only still-to-be handled vessels were in her nasal cavity, and those would require a plastic surgeon. It was over. White returned to the waiting room to alert Caroline's parents that she would wake—and she would heal—and she would grow and play as any little girl. "We have the right to be thankful to the Good Lord," White told them. "And to enjoy our victory."[46]

Some minimal bruising and a long wait for her fine blond hair to grow in were the only side effects of Caroline's surgery. The longest-lasting consequence would be the relationship forged between Caroline and her doctor. White visited her family in Sandusky during summer trips to the Breakers Hotel on Lake Erie. He sent her postcards from Leningrad, and would still be writing about her case near the end of his life. She would speak at his funeral service. It's true that White befriended and was remembered by many of his patients; but Caroline's story was more than one of a surgical intervention. It was a triumph of hope and faith—and it was proof, incontrovertible proof, according to White, that his experimental surgeries were saving little children. That he, Robert White, was saving them. That's what the monkeys were for, he insisted: to be useful in the service of man. The "misguided radicals," as White called PETA, threatened doctors' work to save lives.[47]

Whatever epithets he lobbed at the activists, his principal claim proved more than correct. One by one, labs around the country began feeling the pinch as Newkirk and Pacheco successfully lobbied on behalf of animals. Despite everything White might try to prove, they seemed to be winning.

## THROWING THE GAUNTLET

In May 1983, a month before Caroline's surgery, PETA managed to shut down the US Department of Defense's "wound lab" and successfully lobbied for a ban on the use of cats and dogs in studying gunshot wounds and how they heal. In 1985, they publicized photos of starving animals at City of Hope National Medical Center in Duarte,

California, resulting in the loss of over one million dollars in federal research funding. Both Harvard Medical School and MIT had been forced to cut back on research after new regulations were passed; White—a graduate of Harvard Med—complained that they couldn't procure anything "larger than a rat" (though in fact, lab regulations in Boston were less strict than those in Cambridge).[48]

Relatively few university labs were taken to court by PETA. However, the financial toll and bad press for those that were, not to mention the reticence of funding bodies to raise the ire of activists, meant most labs would rather self-police than end up in PETA's crosshairs. At the same time, certain fringe branches of the animal rights movement had other means of making their presence known—and feared. In 1986, a lab at the University of California, Davis, was vandalized at a cost of $3.5 million. A few months later, an animal rights group called the Band of Mercy stole twenty-eight cats from a lab in Maryland, eleven of which had been infected with *Toxoplasma gondii*, a parasite that causes birth defects in humans, meaning the release of the animals potentially put people (particularly pregnant women and those with immune deficiencies) at risk. Then, the Animal Liberation Front (ALF) attacked California's Riverside Hospital labs, causing half a million in damages and releasing 467 animals, including monkeys being used in a study to improve sight for blind children.[49] These were isolated cases, perpetrated by the few and not the many—and no one had been injured. But bomb scares had begun as well, some carried out by the Animal Rights Militia, a loose band of leaderless activists in the UK who sent letter bombs to researchers as well as major political figures, such as Margaret Thatcher. The militia had cells in the United States as well and took credit for a 1987 arson attack on a lab in California, though they never became as active in the States as they were in the UK. All the same, against the backdrop of Irish Republican Army bombings, which terrorized parts of Ireland and England throughout the 1980s and which had been amply covered by the US media, the threat at least *seemed* very real. Researchers feared disparagement from an angry public on the one hand, and serious injury to life, limb, and property on the other.

Neither the ALF nor PETA sanctioned violence against human life. PETA asserts that its tactics remained firmly rooted in legal action and shaping pop culture—culminating in the 1988 MTV-televised Animal Rights Music Fest, where headliners like the B-52s and Natalie Merchant took the stage to support Ingrid Newkirk as she addressed some 35,000 people in front of the Washington Monument. But whatever their tactics, Robert White considered all antivivisection and animal rights groups guilty of emotional and false propaganda, pulling the strings of congressmen with the "mindless intimidation" of "fanatics."[50] He watched as crowds flocked to the standard-bearers of the movement, and listened to the increasing concerns of his colleagues, who feared their labs might be shut down and their research subjects taken away. At Metro, he had faced no such problems—at least, not yet. The hospital had supported the continued research White and his team were doing with supercooling the primate brain.

In his perfusion experiments, he'd been noticing a troubling coagulopathy, the impaired ability of the blood to coagulate, leading to excessive bleeding (a dangerous problem for any surgery). White theorized that the use of external warming blankets around the *body* of a monkey would insulate it against the hypothermic brain. His team proved that, done successfully, there would be no need for anticoagulant drugs; the brain could be quickly cooled without any harm to the body itself.

Additionally, however, White was continuing to investigate the monkey brain itself—particularly the hemispheres, work he'd begun shortly after the head transplant in 1970. Collaborating with the

Division of Endocrinology and the Department of Obstetrics and Gynecology at University Hospital in Cleveland, White's team "split" a monkey's brain vascularly, opening the monkey's cranium and separating the two hemispheres so that they had separate blood supplies. Then, with the endocrine team, they introduced insulin, estrogen, progesterone, and even gonadal steroids into one half of the brain. Essentially, White had just doubled the utility of a single monkey, which acted both as experimental animal and control group: one side of its brain without the added chemicals and hormones, and one side stimulated by them.[51] White's most significant publications on these matters would open up research into why and how the human brain responds to different stimulus, with implications for better pharmaceutical and surgical outcomes. He had tinkered with his protocols until they were, to his mind, perfected for the primate. The goal was now to scale up the models for humans, something he would spend the next decade pursuing. After all, for White, that was the whole *point* of animal research: you perfect the technique in animals so that by the time you perform the surgery on human beings, you are no longer "experimenting." For a man like White, PETA—and Newkirk in particular—offended against the very lives he saved.

White felt that animal activists cared more for laboratory rats than for Caroline—who had just done a class project on Dr. White's work, complete with an essay about her ordeal and photos of the two of them together. White had spent fifteen months working on animals in order to perform her surgery. For White, those experiments meant the difference between a surgery that worked and a child in the grave. He wasn't going to let PETA's claims go unanswered.[52] And so, in March 1988, White composed an article for *Reader's Digest* titled "The Facts about Animal Research." He had chosen *Reader's Digest* because it turned up in homes across the country, stacked next to TV tables and in lavatories, dog-eared at bedsides and perused at breakfast like the morning paper—it was a way to reach a large and diverse audience of "average" people.

"Do we want to wipe out leukemia? Alzheimer's? AIDS?" White's article asked. He had complained before about what he considered the dangerous and backward-looking opinions of individual animal rights activists, like Catherine Roberts, but now he was taking on the organizations themselves. White had no objection to safeguards; he wanted "healthy research subjects that are not the victims of physical or emotional stress."[53] But, he claimed, PETA aimed to halt scientific progress by making it impossible to do medical research. Did the public want to return to the dark ages of medicine, when children died or were crippled by diseases now eradicated? Of course not. White concluded his article with a call to action of his own, telling readers to write to their congressional representatives and oppose "the bureaucratic regulation[s] that already have added far too much to the cost of medical research."[54] Do it for science, he encouraged. Do it for the *children*.

White's article would act as the opening shot in a new and bitter contest. He'd expected a reaction; that had been the point, really. He did not expect his enemy to be so mobilized, or so militant, in their response. When the March issue of *Reader's Digest* appeared, animal rights activists from around the country descended on the magazine's headquarters in Pleasantville, New York. They demanded justice; they wanted the article retracted and apologies made. At least forty members of PETA joined a press conference during the protest to list their grievances; there was also a wreath-laying ceremony for the animals that died in White's experiments, and a reading of letters of support for animal rights from physicians, senators, and others who had been unable to attend.[55]

Interestingly, White had not—up until now—been a principal

1

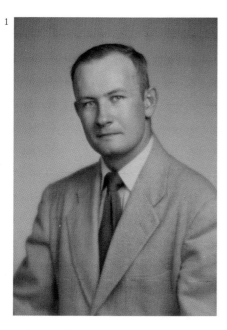

2

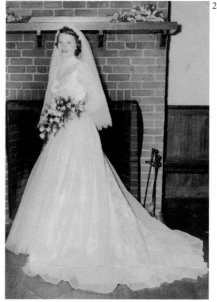

Robert White transferred to Harvard Medical School on a scholarship just months before Joseph Murray performed the world's first successful kidney transplant at Boston's Peter Bent Brigham Hospital in 1954. The triumph would spark the young surgeon-scientist's interest in organ transplant.

White was a multihyphenate talent, but he was also playful and charming, gladly joining med school classmates on a jaunt to New York, where they chatted up Rockettes outside Radio City Music Hall. Still, his first love was surgery. He even met his wife, Patricia, a nurse, in the middle of an appendectomy, later claiming that he "fell in love over an operating table."

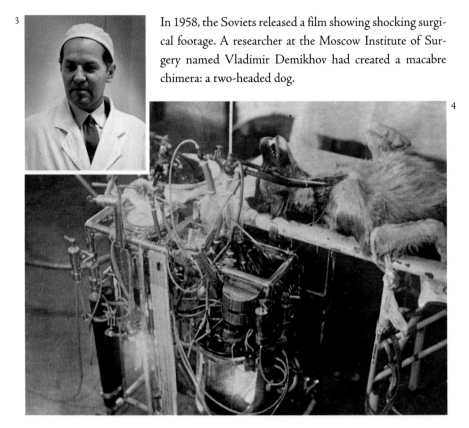

3  In 1958, the Soviets released a film showing shocking surgical footage. A researcher at the Moscow Institute of Surgery named Vladimir Demikhov had created a macabre chimera: a two-headed dog.

4

Demikhov had attached a puppy's head and forelimbs to the back of an adult dog, joining the two animals' vascular systems. Once the anesthesia wore off, both dogs awoke and could breathe, eat, and drink. The experiment demonstrated the possibility of providing a living head with an entirely new body.

5  Demikhov, who'd been conducting life-and-death experiments on stray animals since the age of twenty-one, had performed the surgery using his own tools and modified life-support machines. He managed to reattach the vascular system so quickly that the dogs did not suffer critical brain damage.

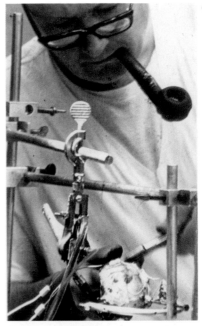

Spurred on by the achievements of his Russian rival, White began his own experiments in his newly renovated Brain Research Lab in downtown Cleveland. His goal: to keep a brain alive outside its body and to demonstrate that it could still "think."

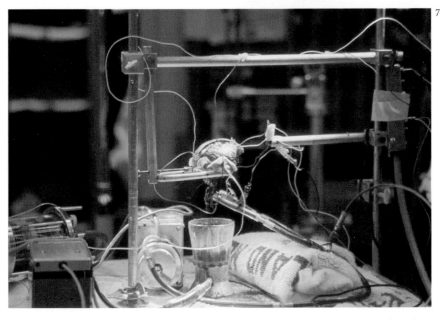

By using perfusion (a cooling process that reduces the brain's need for oxygen), White successfully isolated the brain of a monkey and recorded EEG activity, proving that the brain remained alive. White's new technique of cooling the brain so that it entered a type of protective hibernation would soon appear in operating rooms around the country, preventing catastrophic brain damage and saving lives.

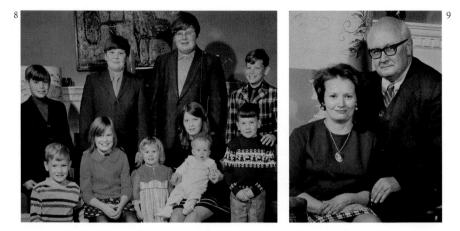

White's neighbors knew him as the devoted head of neurosurgery at Cleveland Metropolitan General, a committed Catholic, and a doting family man. He and Patricia raised ten children in their Shaker Heights home: Bobby, Chris, Patty, Michael, Danny, Pam, Jim, Richard, Marguerite, and Ruth.

As part of his official duties at Metro General, White played host to visiting delegations from Russia and Latvia—a rare honor during the Cold War. White hoped the Russians might reciprocate with an invitation to travel to Moscow and learn from Vladimir Demikhov—but the trip wouldn't prove as beneficial as he'd wished. White had already eclipsed his rival.

By March of 1970, White was ready to perform his first brain transplant. He intended to remove one monkey's head and replace it with the head of another, using the same technique as in the isolation surgeries—except this time the head would be attached to a new body. With the head intact, White would be able to monitor the monkey's response when it awoke.

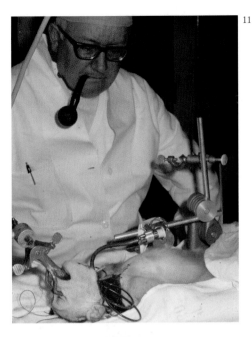

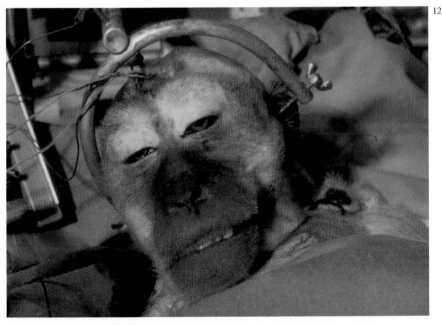

Upon waking, the monkey followed White with its eyes, wrinkled its nose, and even tried to bite. White had proven that, though no longer on its original body, the monkey's brain was living and aware of its surroundings. Because the spine had been severed, the body couldn't move—the monkey was paralyzed from the neck down. The newspapers began to call him "Dr. Frankenstein."

13

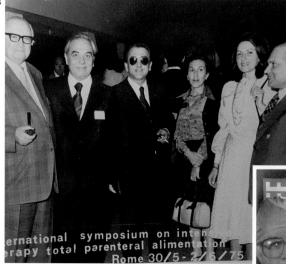

*Below*: Not content to speak only among professional colleagues, White courted public attention, appearing in national and local newspapers, magazines, and even live comedy broadcasts.

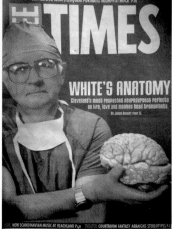

14

ART: SEYDOU KEITA'S ELOQUENT PORTRAITS TRIUMPH AT MOCA P.26

**TIMES**

**WHITE'S ANATOMY**
Cleveland's most respected neurosurgeon reflects on life, love and monkey head transplants.
By James Renner, Page 15

MUSIC: NEW SCANDINAVIAN MUSIC AT BEACHLAND P.40   THEATER: COURTROOM FANTASY ARRAIGNS STEREOTYPES P.22

*Above*: In the years following the successful head transplant, White traveled extensively, speaking at conferences (such as this one in Italy) about the possibilities for extending human life. If the body itself were dying, he argued, the brain and soul could be preserved by moving them to a new body's life support.

15

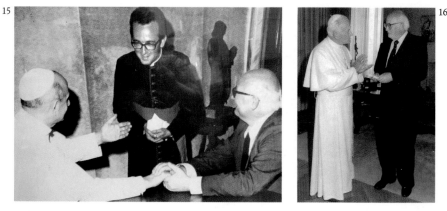

16

White considered both Pope Paul VI and Pope John Paul II his friends and was tapped to head the latter's Vatican Council on Bioethics. His efforts would help change the Church's definition of "death" to be synonymous with "brain death," allowing the harvesting of organs before body functions shut down—and making it ethically (and legally) possible to one day attempt a head transplant on a human.

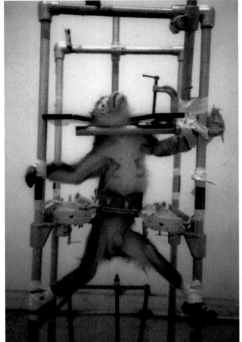

## 17

In September 1981, an image of a shackled rhesus monkey appeared in papers across the United States. The photo came from a lab in Silver Spring, Maryland, which a year-old animal rights group called PETA had gotten raided on the grounds of animal cruelty. The ensuing high-profile case brought medical ethics into the national spotlight and raised the alarm for scientific researchers using lab animals—including one Dr. Robert White.

## 18

White quickly became one of PETA's enemies; his articles attacking the organization earned him the nickname "Dr. Butcher." Far from objecting, he reveled in such comparisons, even posing for a photo dressed as Dr. Frankenstein.

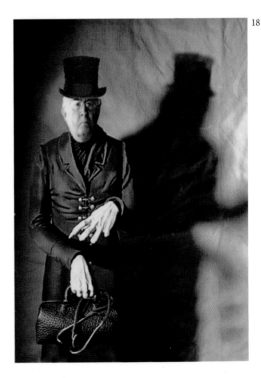

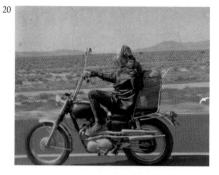

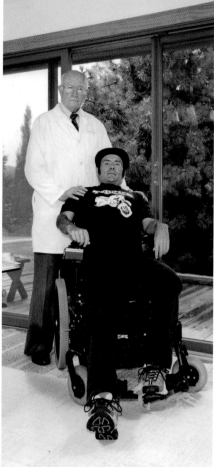

As the new millennium approached, White was ready to proceed with what he now called the full-body transplant. But first he needed to find the perfect patient: a man every bit as daring as himself. Fate led him to Craig Vetovitz, an avid race-car enthusiast, inventor, and entrepreneur, seen here on a cross-country motorcycle trek months prior to the accident that left him paralyzed. *Right:* White and Vetovitz made the case for the full-body transplant on national TV—but the White surgery was not to be. In the former Soviet Union, there was interest but no funding; in the United States, there was money to be had but no support.

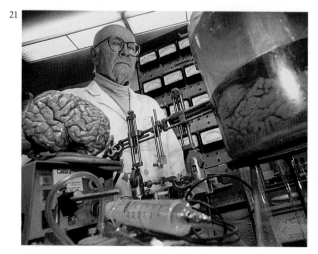

Dr. Robert White's revolutionary work in hypothermia would almost win him the Nobel Prize and his advocacy shaped our modern ethics of brain death. But he remains best remembered not as Humble Bob but as Dr. Butcher, a man whose life ambition was to transplant the human soul.

target for PETA. "I don't know that he was important to us," Newkirk would later say, until he made himself "a very visible part of the problem we were trying to combat."[56] Once White had ensured that PETA took notice, Newkirk explained, PETA felt an obligation to challenge him. He was, in her opinion, a textbook example of experimentation's worst failings—a moral failing, in fact. That he could, "without compunction," cut off the heads of living animals, with all those nerve centers firing, "was all the information we needed."[57] Newkirk called White's work barbaric, comparing it to the torture of the Dark Ages and even to the traffic in human slaves. "The biggest cruelties in our society are those that go on behind closed doors," she argued. "It was just a cosmic wink ago . . . when Africans were plucked from their homelands as chimpanzees are today."[58] People must wake up to these horrors, she insisted. It is our "biggest failing" as a human species that "we like to be led by experts"—experts like Robert White, who "didn't think anyone could touch him."[59]

The White clan in Shaker Heights had shrunk over the years. Of the children, only Ruth remained living at home, with Marguerite popping in for visits, and sometimes Jimmy, who was taking classes at Cleveland State. Most of the time, however, it was just Patricia, Robert, and their youngest, and when the phone rang, no one thought twice about answering.

First, a pause. Then an unfamiliar voice growled into the receiver: "We want to talk to the Butcher." *The who?* Patricia slammed the phone down. But they called back. And they would keep calling. The activists had White's number. His secretary at Metro received calls, too. "Where is Dr. Butcher?" they asked. Sometimes they said worse. Where is the murderer of monkeys, the man who defends his acts of terror against sentient animals? Soon, the post began bringing letters. Flat, white envelopes could not be bombs, but their contents were often laced with verbal threats, and White couldn't afford to take chances. Dr. Andor Sebestény, an animal researcher at the Imperial Cancer Research Fund in the UK, had recently narrowly missed being killed by a car bomb for his work on test animals.[60] White dutifully called the police to report the calls and letters, and became more careful about who answered the telephone.

At least three bomb threats would be made against White by the end of the year, and both the local police and the FBI were brought in to protect his family (as was, for reasons no one seems clear about, the Secret Service).[61] And yet what they offered seemed mainly a show of support rather than a show of force. It barely changed the family's daily routines, and White's wife, Patricia—unflappable as always— remained unruffled by the occasional extra bodies checking in. Even so, some threats became acts.

Protestors broke into a lab at the medical school, mistaking it for White's, and destroyed it; someone tracked White to Metro, intent on doing him harm, but was stopped by police.[62] Getting to and from work became an ordeal of the first order, involving hired cars—no more taking the bus. But White refused to sit at home while his lab remained open. He had to test new advances in supercooling techniques to prevent the formation of ice crystals in the brain. The preparations allowed for long-term storage of (monkey) brains on ice, preserved for White's future use as living experimental subjects. But it also held promise for other things, like the long-term storage of heads for body transplants (which likely explains why cryonics occasionally references White's work). PETA would not cow Dr. White. He went about his life as usual, and continued to win awards, including National Health Professional of the Year in 1988. White was invited to an honor ceremony hosted by the Cleveland Visiting Nursing Association, and his critics determined to make their voices heard, even as he accepted the award.

Dressed in a suit and tie, White climbed into the back seat of the hired car—alone. The ceremony where he planned to accept his award was taking place at a local conference center. His very presence meant a need for increased security; everyone expected picketers, and perhaps even the media, to turn up. No one expected them to come dressed as giant monkeys.

Like a scene from *Planet of the Apes*, men and women in gorilla suits surrounded the car on three sides as it approached the conference center. The driver crept forward carefully as the shouting, whooping crowd pressed against and rocked the vehicle. White made a joke about the costumes, but no one could relax until the gates to the facility were closed behind them.[63] Exiting the car, White could see the protestors still; they clung to the bars of the fence, shaking and rattling them.[64] It's possible they rattled *him* as well, but he entered the hall with good grace. He no doubt thought the rest of the dinner would pass in peace, but he had underestimated the commitment, and theatricality, of his rivals.

Servers swanned about linen-clad tables, and guests toasted with their wineglasses over an excellent meal. As platters were cleared away, the association president rose to give opening remarks, praising White's service to the field, his work as a surgeon, and his value to the medical community. Would he step to the platform and be honored? White rose from his seat, prepared to deliver a short acceptance speech, when a sudden movement rippled across the crowd. Against a background of confused murmurs, a woman in evening attire marched through the room, carrying an unmarked bag. She shouted White's name and threw something heavy, round, and dripping at the stage. It rolled to one side upon landing: a plastic human head, complete with fake blood and gore. The dinner guests nearest the stage looked on, aghast. Security apprehended the woman (who claimed affiliation with PETA), but her accusations rang through the hall: Dr. Butcher didn't deserve any awards. He was the embodiment of hubris, a Frankenstein who cared nothing for the suffering he caused the animals in his lab.

"I'm saddened a bit this evening," White said when he was at last permitted to give his remarks; the head had been gathered up as evidence and removed. "Because I must apologize. It is really so inappropriate that this magnificent banquet should have been interrupted, or indeed as we approached it, [that] we should have been faced with pickets."[65] The measured tone revealed no nerves, no sense of anger at the events. *In fact*, he continued, "I would have been far happier if they had come forward at one of our institutions." He thanked the association for the honor, suggesting at the end of his speech that his satisfaction at receiving it had been tempered only by the fact that his presence had caused some "to be inconvenienced."[66] Attendees would later recount his charm, his unruffled behavior, and his courtesy to those upset by what had happened. No one could deny that the surgeon had nerves of steel.

As ever, he presented an image of perfect composure, but on some level he seemed to take enjoyment from the whole affair. White would come to describe the experience as "one of the most outlandish and at points entertaining things I have ever been in on."[67] And eleven months later, White would face down PETA in a televised public event.

February 10, 1989: A fresh blanket of snow covered the grimed sidewalks downtown, where the City Club of Cleveland had been a fixture since 1912. Located in an imposing Progressive Era building on Euclid Avenue (once known as "millionaires' row"), the home of civic debate offered space for discussion "to help democracy thrive." The stage had been prepared that frigid Friday evening with two podiums, and a chair at each. White sat roughly six feet from Ingrid Newkirk, whom he considered his chief antagonist (whether that was true or not).[68] He had been invited not by Newkirk herself, but by the City Club, which wanted to air the debate on local TV channels as a form of civic outreach. White had come not only to defend himself, but also to advocate for his entire profession—even scientific progress itself.

The audience filed in, filling the room to the back, where cameras waited to capture what happened next. The master of ceremonies stood between the adversaries, red curtain and American flag ruffling with the central heating. The emcee gave the introductions, and the subject of the debate: Should animal experiments be permitted to continue? Then he signaled for Newkirk to take the mic.

In a soft beige suit, and in an equally soft but confident voice, Newkirk began reading from a series of note cards. Animals, she told the audience, had a nervous system like any human; "the suffering they endure is not only physical but psychological . . . they feel pain, fear, and loneliness as we do."[69] She compared the plight of research animals to the fight for rights—not for racial minorities this time, but for those with disabilities or mental health concerns. If you experiment on an animal just because it is not as intellectually developed as an adult human, what does that say of your feelings toward those less intellectual than yourself? Researchers "take apart animals for show," she claimed. There was no lasting benefit to what White and his colleagues did, nothing that could not be done in better and more humane ways, such as using human cells and tissue or computer modeling. "You are torturing animals merely to collect useless data," she claimed, "killing them only to prove what you have the skill and the power to do."[70]

The room shifted uncomfortably as Newkirk resumed her seat. The emcee signaled to White, but when he stepped to his podium, he remained silent for a long moment. His gaze traveled about the room; he knew many of these people, educated and civic-minded and curious. This was his city. At last, White's eyes fell upon a figure sitting primly near the front, and he smiled at her: *Not yet*. Then he straightened his suit, adjusted his rectangular frames, and spoke without notes (though not without advance preparation).

"I rise as a representative of the medical profession," he began in a voice both sonorous and pleasant. "What you have heard today from Ms. Newkirk is *anti-science*. She is not a vet, a physician, or a lab investigator," and yet she stood there making grand scientific claims.[71] "You have been told," he went on, "that a baby rat equals a human baby"; in other words, that all lives are the same, that there can be no difference, no gradation, from the least to the greatest being on this planet. White's voice lifted ever so slightly. *Everyone* agrees that animals must have the very best care, he insisted, then wagged his finger at the audience. "Ms. Newkirk is not arguing for better care"; what she wanted was to abolish all scientific research involving animals. White leaned across the podium, his face open, friendly, as if asking those gathered to see the greater sense. *Listen*, he seemed to say, *and I will tell you what it means to be a surgeon scientist.*

"I just took care of a two-year-old child with a tumor. And yesterday, I was operating deep in a woman's brain." White stood straighter, his voice growing stronger with emotion. "How many of you sitting out there had open heart surgery? Hmm? How many of you would like to have had it done for the first time?"[72] Out before him, the audience had moved almost imperceptibly forward. White threw his shoulders back, head up, eyes alight. Animal experiments made it possible, White went on, for surgeons to save *your* lives, and the lives of your loved ones. He'd made it local, personal. And he rebuked Newkirk's claims that such strides could have been made without animal models. Activists had suggested that animal rights and human rights were the same; they wanted to join forces with the civil rights movement. But the human was more than animal, and equating the two was not only wrong, it was *dangerous*. White broke his gaze to reach inside his breast pocket. Carefully, he unfolded a press release from 1933 and proceeded to read aloud the German policy to end vivisection and to raise the status of all animals almost to that of humans. The anti-animal-experiment policy had been signed by Adolf Hitler. He had "saved" animals from experimentation, all right, but only by performing grisly medical experiments upon Jewish men, women, and children.

An unsettled hush fell upon the room, and White laid the paper aside. "I really don't know what else to say," he added. "This has not been an easy year for me." Voice lowered, and now seeming to shrink back into himself, White told the audience of the threats made against his family. "Why should I stand before you when my life is being threatened by these people?" he asked, pointedly not looking at Ingrid Newkirk. Why hadn't he stayed at home, kept his profile low, gone away quietly? "Because," he answered, "unless we continue to support science, more people will die. Tens of thousands of young people will die. Can you accept that?"[73] In silence, White signaled to a seated woman. "In many ways the PETA people are wonderful people religiously committed to what they believe," White said, but in his view, they put animals above humans; "this"—White smiled gently—"I cannot do." He reached a hand to the woman. "I would like to introduce a guest. Carla, could you stand?" She smiled nervously and greeted the crowd. Without the monkey experiments, White explained, Carla would not be here. Without the monkeys, *Caroline* would not be here, either—nor would many, many of White's other patients, young and old. Carla happily told the assembly that she owed her life to White. It served as his closing remark.

Ingrid Newkirk knew she was up against long odds in Cleveland, Dr. White's home turf. She admitted that she didn't think she could "win" against him there, but that she owed it to the cause of animal rights to meet his challenge. It wasn't that she found White charismatic, exactly; "I remember him being quiet, cutting, and self-assured," she said, "a pudgy white blob of confidence."[74] Though White had clearly commanded the room during the presentation, in a Q&A session that followed, he shot down the query of a young medical student who showed some support for Newkirk's ideas by telling him, "You are not in the position to question science."[75] Still, the evening was, Newkirk later admitted, a memorable occasion. It demonstrated how thoroughly White believed himself to be in the right; he wasn't experimenting on animals out of malice, after all. He just didn't think animals would ever be as important as people; their welfare simply didn't compete. But the event proved something else, as well; White felt that if PETA could do so-called publicity stunts, then so could he.[76]

Science has long relied on public performance. Early experiments in electricity took place in large public squares, almost like carnival entertainment—and in more recent memory, the first to get their work into the public forum got to claim the discovery of double-helix DNA, with the credit going to Watson and Crick rather than to Rosalind Franklin, without whose X-ray diffraction images, no discovery would have been possible. The scientist does not *have* to be a showman, a darling of the media, like South Africa's Christiaan Barnard. But it helps. White already knew that; he had been practicing his charm since long before PETA darkened his laboratory door. He had even once performed a minor miracle on an old dog to prove a point to his priest.

This "miracle" had taken place years earlier, slightly prior to the monkey head transplant, back when White was still keen to "prove" that brain death equaled actual death. Some few hours before noon, White had had his technician anesthetize the dog; he then hooked it up to cooling technology (the same he would have used on Caroline, if it had come to that) and slowly cooled the body to 10 degrees Celsius. The dog's limbs went stiff as a board, stuck out rigid on the table. But White hadn't finished. He tapped the dog's primary vessels and drained all the blood away.[77] Slowly, a containment unit filled with the precious liquid, dark sanguine, as the nearly frozen dog's heart came to a stop. Preparations complete, White opened the lab door.

"Come in, Father," he said to the Jesuit priest. "It's lunchtime." White pulled chairs around the operating table—the same table where the bloodless frozen dog still lay—and laid down a picnic cloth. He'd brought sandwiches. He invited the priest to join him, but the poor man waved away White's request with a sour face.[78] White and the other team members began to eat, and between bites, White gave the priest a calculated look. "Father, tell me—is this dog dead?" he asked. The priest, who kept his distance from the animal, cleared his throat from where he stood near the door. Yes, the priest agreed. Of course it was dead. White smiled in deep satisfaction. Then he swept away the picnic debris, sent the dog's blood swirling back into its veins, warmed its body, and restarted its heart. In just under an hour, the mongrel opened its eyes, got up from the table, and walked about the room, to the combined horror and delight of the good father. "Maybe like Christ," White said with a mischievous wink, "dead and revived?"[79]

Was the dog dead? It depended upon your definition. Prior to White's founding of the Vatican bioethics council, the Church maintained that to have no blood, breath, or heartbeat—to be so cold that to bare fingers, the skin felt cool on contact, that limbs and soft tissue grew rigid and without sensation—was to be most assuredly deceased. But White had not killed the dog. He had *suspended it*. By supercooling the animal's body and brain, he put its life in limbo. Was the dog alive? White told the surprised priest, "You say the body functions must collapse at death. I say that if the brain signal collapses, then the human is dead, though the body may continue on."[80] In other words, the look of a body didn't matter if the brain lived; brain death should be the only death. White had used the dog as experiment, as prop—to prove a point.

PETA would fail to shut down Dr. White. They wouldn't bring him to court, either. For Newkirk, chasing White was unlikely to prove advantageous; he was only one man. They did far better work fighting the NIH for control of the Silver Spring monkeys, a battle that ended up in the highest court in the land. They would also grow very effective at lobbying, and through their campaigns would even cause NASA to pull out of the Bion mission experiments—a joint US, French, and Russian program in the early 1990s that planned to implant electrodes into the bodies of space-destined monkeys. Directly or indirectly, PETA had introduced changes in animal welfare by mobilizing the public—and by making funding bodies and universities shy away from the animal rights controversy.

White had grown used to asking hard questions of the public and fighting like hell to achieve his ends. He'd published in esteemed academic journals and written for mass media; he'd appeared on television and debated public figureheads. In short, though White may attack PETA, he operated in much the same way Ingrid Newkirk had done, and with the same level of conviction. Newkirk pointed to White's blind spots: White pointed right back. For White, life—human life—meant everything. It meant that so long as he worked to preserve this end, God was with him, too. "There are immense resources behind me," he had told *People* magazine, divine resources, and he believed it still.

He was playing God *for* God; he would be God's own hands. He had faced down the medical establishment, he had overcome the doubts of his chosen church, and he had faced his keenest adversaries without giving ground. The way must surely now be clear for the future of transplant. The questions were no longer *if* and *how* but *whom* and *when*. The first successful transplants of hearts and kidneys had been acts of desperation—the last effort to stall death's slow walk across the human body. But the body-brain transplant meant far more than replumbing spare parts. This was treading into the sacred ground of identity—and Dr. White was ready. He could do nothing more with monkeys to further his aims; like Christiaan Barnard or Joseph Murray before him, he needed to perform the surgery on a human being for it to truly set precedent. And since the experiment would involve consenting humans, this next step technically wouldn't fall under PETA's purview at all. The question was, would any patient willingly agree to take the risk?

# Chapter 8

# THE PERFECT PATIENT

*W*hite's office tended toward overstuffed. A bust of Lenin and several partial models of the human brain stood guard over the usual desk detritus of files, case notes, and research articles. A tower of newspapers leaned in the corner, along with *A Literary History of Russia,* a biography of Saint Francis of Assisi, and *How to Deep-Freeze a Mammoth.*[1] There were filing cabinets, too. And boxes. Lots of boxes. White thumbed through files in a bid at organization, picking out the one on the Sam Sheppard trial. The neurosurgeon had been exonerated after serving ten years in prison for murdering his wife; his son later sued the state of Ohio for wrongful imprisonment. White had taken the stand during that later civil trial. It wasn't the first time he'd been called as an expert witness, but it still had a certain buzz to it, especially after Harrison Ford played a fictionalized version of Sam Sheppard in *The Fugitive.* Sheppard originally claimed to have injured himself in a struggle with an intruder—and that this intruder had murdered his wife. X-rays were provided in the trial, as proof. White, however, testified that the X-rays did not belong to Sheppard. He went so far as to suggest that Sheppard forged them to provide himself an alibi. The Sheppard family lawyer angrily shouted that no one need listen to this, this *Frankenstein* . . . but ultimately, White's expert opinion won out.[2]

Then there was the Cold War–era letter from the State Department. An American Marine, on a delegation to Russia, had fallen four stories from a window onto the street below. The State Department had called Dr. White immediately; how were they to remove the man? Sending in military helicopters for transport could incite a war. Dr. White had helped arrange for a plane from Helsinki, in neutral Finland, to pick up the wounded soldier and fly him to a base in Germany. White had asked the government to send Russia a collection of microsurgical textbooks and journals, which were barred from export to the Communist country, in thanks. He saw those textbooks in a Russian library years later.[3] Couldn't part with that letter, either. In fact, White didn't want to part with any of it. The lab, the operating room, the years of work at Metro—they were White's whole life.[4] But the time was coming. By the end of the decade, on the eve of a new millennium, he would be asked to move on. To *retire*.

It began with hints and questions. When would White move to that beach house Patricia had always wanted? She had been looking at listings in Geneva-on-the-Lake, a charming community along Lake Erie that had the aura of a seaside town, with arcades and boardwalks. The big rambling house in Shaker Heights was too large and too quiet for her; most of the children had moved far away, scattered from Arizona to Minnesota. Two could be very happy in a cottage on a lake, she insisted. White looked over the housing brochures, thumbing the glossy photos, but his heart wasn't in it. He'd spent the better part of the last decade performing batteries of experiments, improving even the smallest details of brain isolation, cooling, and storage. *What if*, he asked, a child whose body had been eaten up by disease could be saved by separating her head from her ailing body?[5] How could he think of retirement now, when he was so close to perfecting the human trial transplant surgery? He would not go willingly. But he might not have much choice.

Metro was changing fast. White's old allies and friends had gone. Frank E. Nulsen, who'd originally brought White on board, had passed away in 1994, and Maurice Albin had moved on to a post at the University of Michigan. Both White and Albin had appeared as characters in Peter Niesewand's 1982 espionage novel, *Fall Back*—which includes, unsurprisingly, a head transplant. They had shared a lot more than that little nugget of fame, but they no longer shared the operating room. In place of familiar faces were new and younger doctors and department heads, all interested in expanding the hospital as a trauma center . . . and not so interested in the experimental brain work taking up an entire floor. Nicholas Regush of ABC had produced a story for *World News Tonight* with Peter Jennings about White's monkey transplant surgery; he caught up with White again for an opinion piece, only *this* time he asked White if he was just "pushing the envelope." After all, taking heads off at his age wasn't "the most gracious way to top off a long career."[6] White responded testily, "Just because I'm older now, does that mean I have to stop imagining how I can contribute to science?"[7] If *I* don't do it, went White's logic, then someone else will. And they wouldn't do it as well.

Murray's kidney transplant, Barnard's heart transplant, and many more "firsts" that followed . . . all that they'd achieved had also once been called impossible. There were two things that had made those early surgeries successful: the first was experimentation and the second was public consent. A "total body transplant," as White now called the surgery, was one and the same. Having already struggled with his public image due to his fights against PETA, White feared a wave of popular rejection would hobble his attempts. But he could no longer proceed with caution. His office might soon be someone else's, his boxes relegated to an emeritus workspace down the hall. He might be running out of time, and yet the mid- to late 1990s also offered the greatest acceptance of brain death, organ donation, and organ harvesting yet known. Once taboo, the idea of a dead brain in a live body had taken hold in the public consciousness. If ever there was going to be a time for the "White Surgery," as he sometimes liked to call it, that time was *now*.

## THE WHITE PRINCIPLE

The Uniform Determination of Death Act (UDDA) had finally been instituted in the United States in 1981 to standardize brain death criteria. White very proudly asserted that he'd "designed" this definition of brain death; his work did have bearings upon the definition, and certainly mattered from the Vatican's point of view, but the act's exact wording had been determined by the National Conference of Commissioners on Uniform State Laws, in cooperation with the American Medical Association, the American Bar Association, and the President's Commission for the Study of Ethical Problems in Medicine and Biomedical and Behavioral Research.[8] UDDA held that though existing common law defined death as a total failure of the cardiorespiratory system, common law would have to be extended to include patients on respirators who had irreversible loss of all brain function. If a patient's heart and lungs ceased to operate, the patient had died (by this definition); if the patient were kept alive via a ventilator and feeding tubes, but "the entire brain" had ceased to function, then he or she was *also* considered dead under the law.[9] Life support could be removed—and with it, the organs for donation.[10] In a sense, the legalities just confirmed what those first jurors had decided in the Tucker case. To no one's surprise, White extrapolated from this definition to defend his belief that all of the so-called human element resided in the brain as a soul.

The *New York Times* once asked White how much a soul weighed. Ever since the seventeenth century—going back at least to René Descartes, who believed the soul must live in the pituitary gland—scientists and polymaths had tried in vain to discover the physical soul. If such a thing really existed, the *Times* suggested, then it would surely be measurable: it would have a structure and neural connections.[11] White had answered, rather slyly, that you cannot see gravity, only its effects, and yet it exists. The soul need not have a physical structure that we can detect, he explained, because it existed in "the fourth dimension."[12] We must look beyond a mind-body relationship, he insisted, and understand the more philosophically complex mind-soul-body relationship. The physical, three-dimensional body-brain, White explained, "*faces*" the soul. To access it, "you have to cross the physical space, from the third, to the fourth dimension."[13] It requires a great deal of mental acrobatics to visualize this, a kind of multidimensional Venn diagram, with the brain and body on one plane, intersected on another by a soul that bridges the invisible distance between brain and mind. This strange metaphysical connection, in all its complexity, he called "The White Principle."

Science demanded proof. Catholicism required faith. White never considered them opposed, but as he aged, he went further in trying to unite them through his own philosophical doctrine. Since he never considered monkeys to be en-souled, a primate head transplant hadn't required these complicated philosophical considerations. But if White maintained that a physical human brain also contained the nonmaterial soul, this raised several serious questions. The physical properties of the brain were not equal to the soul; yet the brain housed the soul and served in some sense as its retaining organ. So *how much of the brain did you need?* The PhD monkeys (macaques trained by White's lab to test learning and function before and after hemispherectomy) retained their personalities and memories in *half* a brain. There was even a young woman at Johns Hopkins whose temporal lobes had been destroyed and her brain's language center lost who had somehow made a full recovery.[14] Then there were his own patients, including one White had assumed would never wake from coma; half his brain had liquefied from impact trauma and had to be siphoned out, yet he relearned to speak and even to play chess again.[15]

Somehow, White reasoned, making the container smaller did not hew away at the soul inside; it simply flowed into the remaining spaces, took up residence there, and thrived. The soul must suffuse the very cells of the brain, White decided, but could move easily between them. "I could argue that the soul is connected to a special part of what I call the *cell genetic strand*," he explained to a friend, German journalist Christian Jungblut. "The connection occurs in the genetic strand of the first cell, the zygote, but only to a specific part—just the segment of DNA that contains information for building the brain."[16] It remained an open sort of theory, a working hypothesis. But in his own mind, White needed to be certain that a human head transplant preserved the God-created immortality that differentiated humans from all other animals. Without weight, without permanent ties to the body, fluid enough to take space in any part of a living brain, the soul traveled light. It could make the short journey from one body to the next.

But the question remained: Who would want to try it? On White's desk lay folded diagrams modeling the procedure, demonstrating where the screws and plates and stitches would be following the surgery. The pictured human being in the diagram had a generic look: a blond, placid-faced Ken-doll sort of man. But White's favorite fantasy patient was British physicist Stephen Hawking. Diagnosed with amyotrophic lateral sclerosis (ALS, often called Lou Gehrig's disease) at twenty-two, Hawking suffered a slow degeneration of motor function until his brain no longer controlled any voluntary muscles in his body. He appeared in films and on television, wrote books, and launched some of the greatest debates of our age concerning physics, science, and the human spirit—including ability, disability, and what it means to have a body in the first place. More than anyone on this planet, Hawking was a *brain*, a brilliant mind housed in an organic life-support system that provided little more than the blood flow, air flow, and electrical pulses to keep the lights on. White went so far as to call him a "head on a computer." If anyone proved there were reasons to preserve the brain when the body ceased to be useful, Hawking was it.[17] For Hawking (and paralyzed actor Christopher Reeve, another of White's favorite examples), the organs of the body would eventually collapse, but they could live on—perhaps indefinitely—in new bodies.[18]

Of course, Stephen Hawking did not believe in eternal souls, nor did he seem interested in being removed from his present body. Hawking wasn't *confined* by his condition. He was *defined* by it. "My disabilities have not been a significant handicap," he wrote in *Science Digest* in 1984; in fact, "they have shielded me" from the demands on a body— the expectations of doing and moving that burden the mobile. White liked the idea of trialing his full-body transplant on Hawking anyway. He especially enjoyed the possibility of proving to Hawking that the physicist had a soul; wouldn't that, White asked, "be a riveting scenario for the world to consider"?[19] But Hawking would never be White's patient. Who, then? What the surgery required was a pioneer just as interested in pushing the envelope as White was himself.

•   •   •

Craig Vetovitz smiled from his wheelchair for Channel 23 News, his newsboy cap firmly in place. The station had come to feature his company, Dynamic Coating, as its "business of the week." Behind him, a race car body hung suspended by pulleys over a gleaming engine. "I loved racing. After the accident, I wanted to stay involved," he explained.[20] The camera cut to his right hand, resting on the chair's navigation system. Lacking fine motor control, Vetovitz would never again sit behind the wheel of a race car, but that hadn't stopped him from leaving his mark on the track. Vetovitz developed a polymer coating for engine parts to reduce friction, allowing cars to go faster without breaking down. The coating, thinner than Teflon and resistant to wearing off, even caught the attention of NASA, which offered him a contract to help them reduce friction in the space shuttle. "The applications are limitless," he said, "and I like testing the limits . . . Being in a wheelchair . . ." He trailed off for a moment before continuing. "It's changed my life, but I basically have to overlook the handicap part."[21] He smiled again at the chassis behind him, sleek in bold racing colors. Not everyone wanted a career surrounded by reminders of what they had been and could now never be. But Craig Vetovitz wasn't everyone.

The accident had happened in 1971. A recent graduate from high school, Vetovitz had just returned from a cross-country motorcycle trek. His streaked blue motorbike, complete with overstuffed camp pack, had traced a route through the great American Southwest, ending at his uncle's home in Michigan. He worked the summer there, and then, on a hot and sticky afternoon, paid a visit to his parents' home not far from Cleveland, Ohio.

The house was built on a hill, and the roofline sloped closer to the ground in the back—just above an inviting swimming pool. The distance made it the perfect platform for diving into the water, even if the roof was a *bit* too high. Vetovitz's grandmother cautioned him not to attempt it, but his first dive went smoothly, a burst of speed and a rush of cold water. He climbed out, dripping and laughing, ready for a second attempt. On the way down, he failed to get his arms out in front of himself to break the surface tension of the water: a minor error, but a devastating one. His head hit the water first, ricocheting back and to the side from velocity and water tension. The quick snap didn't fracture the vertebrae so much as crush them.

When the body goes into shock, it cannot respond to signals from the brain, leading it to shut down. Craig Vetovitz died that day—three times. Paramedics brought him back to life at the scene of the accident, still limp and wet, as his terrified family looked on. They revived him again in the emergency room, and once more when he flatlined on the operating table. He would live, but life would never be the same.

Vetovitz had lost all motor control of his lower body and most physical sensation, too (he retained a slight ticklishness in one foot). He could shrug his shoulders, but his limbs were so rigid that his physicians could not extend his knees or flex his hips on either side. Frozen toes made it difficult to remove his socks and shoes, and his fingers and hands had poor dexterity and were often unresponsive.[22] After his initial recovery and stabilization, myelography (an imaging technique that uses a needle to inject contrast dye into the spinal canal) revealed the worst: a slim, atrophied spinal cord at the C3–C4 vertebrae. Vetovitz was now quadriplegic; he would live the rest of his life in a wheelchair.[23]

C4 quadriplegia is generally considered the most severe level of spinal cord injury. Vetovitz spent over a year and a half in Cleveland's Highland View hospital, some thirteen miles south of Metro, but his physicians were not really working toward full rehabilitation; it simply wasn't possible. Vetovitz considered that giving in. There *must* be better ways, he thought, and decided upon a radical solution. He checked himself out of the hospital and moved into the apartment of a veteran he'd met there who had been a medic. Together, the two constructed braces out of scrap aluminum and worked on muscle building. By strengthening his shoulders, Vetovitz began to have at least some control over his arms. He developed a "writing splint," a stiff, castlike apparatus for his arm and hand, so he could learn to write again. A year later, he enrolled in Cuyahoga Community College. He continued rehabilitation nearby, swimming and working on parallel bars to build muscle tone. He wanted to beat his own paralysis, to thwart it, to *win*.[24] In the meantime, he would steal back as much independence as he could. In 1976, Vetovitz and his father designed a home for Craig and his soon-to-be wife, Susan. Octagonal, at ground level, and with low windows that he could look through (or escape through if there were a fire), the house made the news as a concept-designed halfway house where other people in wheelchairs could live communally.[25] Its circular shape meant Vetovitz could always move forward rather than needing to go backward, his mantra for living.

Vetovitz often bragged that he'd accomplished more from his wheelchair than many others had done with no physical limitations at all. He finished his education, got married, had children, started a business, won research grants from NASA, and traveled extensively, including taking jaunts to New Zealand and Fiji.[26] Though he would never drive a race car or ride a motorcycle again, nor play backyard football with his boys, he refused to stop pushing for new horizons. He began a program to train paralyzed patients to work in his business, demonstrated the use of new wheelchairs (such as the GRIT Freedom Chair, an all-terrain wheelchair originally modeled on a golf cart), and held fund-raisers for kids with spinal injuries at Heath Hill Hospital for Children in Cleveland. "It's not disabilities that make a child or an adult handicapped," Vetovitz said in an interview after a charity event in 1991. "It's other people who do . . . by labeling and categorizing them."[27] But he also knew that most of the children at Heath Hill would not live to be teenagers. Bodies are fragile things, after all. For Craig, it would start with his kidneys. They began to fail.

It had been decades since Joseph Murray performed the first kidney transplant, saving the life of Richard Herrick, and a great deal had changed for the better: improved safety, longer life spans for transplant recipients, greater access to organs. Murray himself had retired from Harvard Medical, and was awarded the Nobel Prize in Physiology/Medicine in 1990. But a kidney transplant would never save Craig Vetovitz. By virtue of his paralysis, he would not be considered a "suitable" candidate.[28] Demand for organs was and continues to be very high; the number of kidneys available each year might reach 16,000—leaving 50,000 people on waiting lists.[29] With the needs of so many to be met, transplant centers look carefully and critically at potential recipients. In order to be considered for a transplant, a patient must be "in good health" apart from their renal disease.[30] We require a constant release of hormones and other chemicals to help the body heal, grow, and regulate. Disruption of those signals responsible for keeping the organs and tissues healthy means the entire system can fail. The kidneys act as canaries in a coal mine; if they fail, other organs will follow, one by one. A spinal cord injury interrupts the brain-to-body-to-brain signals necessary for healing. As a result, very few paralyzed patients are considered for kidney transplants—and if considered, are never given priority. Vetovitz knew he would likely never be placed on a waiting list. But he was prepared to put his life in the hands of an experimental surgeon. Bold, intelligent, and unsinkable, Vetovitz was an inventor himself, ready to take risks, to do the unthinkable. And he didn't have much to lose. He was, at least as far as Robert White was concerned, the perfect patient.

## LIVES WORTH SAVING

Articles featuring White's full-body transplant surgery usually asked teasing questions about ethics and religion. Could it *really* be "okay" to take off someone's head? White's answer remained the same as ever. No, it wasn't unethical; no, it wasn't against the church. The Holy Father himself had no objections. In fact, Pope John Paul II had invited White to join the Pontifical Academy of Sciences—the hallowed building he'd visited in Rome all those years before, white marble shining in the sun—and to advise him personally on matters in bioethics.[31] At the time, the Vatican was principally preoccupied with the start of life and the question of abortion; White thought himself an expert on the other end of things, but much of the conversation—and many of his communications to the academy—still revolved around the ambiguous line between what was life and what was not. For White, it still came down to brain activity.* Again and again, White would maintain that there wasn't a problem with the full-body transplant "from a theological or an ethical point of view" because brain death was real death.[32] To many, however, the words felt hollow, an attempt at justifying Frankenstein-like hubris.

"I wish," Vetovitz told his son Kreg, "that there was a pill you could give people to make them paralyzed for a few months." Nothing long term, but a way to make them see through the eyes of those bound to wheelchairs, to witness firsthand the lack of independence and control.

---

*The idea that life begins at conception is quite new for the Catholic Church, and its stance on abortion is only about 150 years old. In the 1869 document *Apostolicae Sedis Moderationi*, Pope Pius IX declared abortion a type of murder. Before this, a fetus was not considered fully alive until "ensoulment," the point at which it had developed a soul, the timeline for which no one seemed to agree upon. Dr. White's own stance on abortion is unclear.

They would see where the real monstrosity lies. "Let's pretend you're a total quad," Vetovitz told a reporter for *Cleveland Scene* magazine. "And let's say you're real thirsty. You gotta ask somebody to get you a glass of water."[33] Then, after drinking that water, you have to ask someone to help you use the toilet, because after paralysis, messages can no longer pass along the spinal nerves between the bladder and the brain. Paralysis wasn't just about what you couldn't do; it was also about boundaries, and the way your body no longer seemed entirely yours. Vetovitz put it another way: "When you become disabled, you lose all privacy."[34] Someone else had to bathe him, dress him . . . Many patients have to have their bladders emptied via catheter every four to six hours. Vetovitz and his wife had divorced, but she continued to care for him—saving him the embarrassment of having strangers (nurses) or, worse, his own sons do intimate tasks for him.

There were other threats, too: deep vein thrombosis (blood clots) from too little movement; bowel trouble; skin lesions and pressure ulcers that could grow infected and lead to sepsis—the life of a paralyzed person is one of constant vigilance. The body becomes the chief negotiator of all that you do, a thing separate from the mind that no longer controls it. "Everybody always thinks 'oh, what a gross, horrible, mean thing'" performing a head transplant must be, Vetovitz complained.[35] But only because they didn't understand. Vetovitz had risen to the challenge of overcoming the obstacles to living a full life as a C4 quad. But he was injured in 1972. At the time, victims of spinal cord injury could expect to live an average of twenty more years. Doctors originally told him he wouldn't make it to thirty years old—and here he was, in his mid-forties. In the medical sense, Vetovitz had already passed his sell-by date. Time was running out, and all risks became relative.[36] He knew of Dr. White; as a local expert in spinal trauma, White had been sent Vetovitz's X-rays all those years ago, though he could do nothing for Craig's injuries. Vetovitz knew about Dr. White's less orthodox work, too.

Vetovitz's interest in experimental surgery had begun with an effort to raise awareness for stem cell treatments, which weren't yet permitted clinically. He started placing opinion pieces in the local press. Perhaps if he showed that patients were willing to go to extraordinary lengths, he would move hearts—and research review boards. He had already met and spoken to Christopher Reeve, another man bent on finding a cure for spinal injuries—but the cure was slow in coming. If his organs failed, he wouldn't be around to see it.

White's work had been featured on local and national television; he'd said repeatedly that the cephalic transplant surgery performed on monkeys could be scaled up for humans, that a human *could* receive a new body. Vetovitz decided to get in touch, and White was only too happy to meet him. The two men appeared together publicly for the first time in 1996 for a three-minute segment on the tabloid news show *Hard Copy*. In post-production edits, the producers changed the voice-over to introduce the pair as "Dr. Frankenstein and his willing monster." They ran the special on Halloween, denigrating White's research—and Vetovitz's willing sacrifice—to a science fiction sideshow. Furious, Vetovitz shouted down the producers and got them to rerelease an edited version of the program. But it *was* shocking. It *was* hard to believe. "We joked with him," his son Kreg explained. "But Dad was ready. And we got used to the idea. I guess we went from denial to disbelief to curiosity."[37]

For Vetovitz, White's research wasn't macabre; it was noble. He insisted that the surgeon understood what it was like to live life as his patients, that he felt their misery and pain.[38] Most people (including the various interviewers and TV and radio correspondents who covered the story) still thought Vetovitz's willingness to be a guinea pig was foolish and rash. But Vetovitz, pioneering and as brassy as White himself, waved them away. He was perfect for this, he maintained, because "[I don't] give a shit about other people's opinions."[39] White came to Vetovitz's specially designed house in Hinckley, Ohio. The two men stood in the pristine white dining area, looking out sliding doors onto a balcony and a sea of green conifers beyond it. White stood behind his new patient, hands resting on Vetovitz's shoulders, as they looked toward the camera. It would be their official press photo. White spoke in terms of the lives he could save, of the time he could buy for patients. People who had been paralyzed may not have been considered the ideal candidates for organ transplants. But they were human beings with human souls. Weren't their lives worth saving?[40]

White had already been busy developing a scaled-up surgical procedure for use in human beings. He even claimed it would be simpler; after all, the veins and arteries—all the tissues, in fact—would be larger and easier to see and work with. On top of that, White knew the human brain and its electrical responses better than those of monkeys. They would just need fail-safe backup systems, bigger teams, and a bigger operating room. He'd even broken down the cost estimates. The surgery itself would run somewhere between $100,000 and $200,000. Not so expensive in the grand scheme of things, White thought—not when you considered that the cost of a kidney transplant averages $400,000 for time and equipment. But of course, White would also need funds for initial training, trials, and a specialized operating room equipped to perform surgery on two different people, with two different surgical teams working in tandem. There would be aftercare, too, and probably rehabilitation, not to mention antirejection drugs. To do all that, the end cost would no doubt be closer to $4 million. He suspected grants would be in order, just as they had been before, with the monkeys. Perhaps the NIH. *Perhaps.* Convincing hospital ethics committees might be difficult, too, even if there was no federal regulating body.* White and Vetovitz both worried that the surgery might still be considered too taboo.

The year 1998 dawned to a cold January and sizzling political scandal (namely, the president's inappropriate relations with a young intern). But the biggest news for White was of a different sort: his time at Metro was now officially just about up. He would have to retire before the end of 1999. That meant less than two years to lay out the exact parameters for a body transplant for Vetovitz—not much time to find a way of sharing the White Surgery with the world.

Dissection rooms have always been the surgeon's private library. The opening of a cadaver, like the pages of an exclusive book, became a rite of passage for many medical students. White wanted to take his surgery protocol forward. He'd imagined it countless times, lying in bed and visualizing the operation, perfecting it in the private space of his own head. Now he wanted his fingers to follow suit, to cut with a scalpel along the lines indicated in his diagrams. He didn't need monkeys any longer; like his literary counterpart, Dr. Frankenstein, he needed a freshly dead body. The usual cadavers in medical schools are preserved, heavy with the smell of chemical fluids that tinge the flesh and stain tissues until none of the interior parts look quite the way they should, and nothing like they do in textbooks. White needed a body untouched by that process: a fresh cadaver, recently living. Like Joseph Murray before him, who had faced icy roads to reach his own freshly dead cadaver for a test-run kidney transplant just days before Christmas, White put in a request

---

*Unlike pharmaceutical innovation, which is regulated by the FDA, there is no standard federal regulation for surgical procedures. As a result, surgical protocol can vary widely from region to region.

for not one but two suitable "patients" for practice. Meanwhile, he pulled out old notebooks, sketches, and plans from the monkey surgeries. He watched the films of the surgeries, too—grainy, but offering disturbing clarity in full color. The question he needed to answer was this: To scale up the surgery from monkey to man, what needed to change?

White unfolded his work like star charts, mapping the stages from the minute vessels of monkeys onto the anatomy of human bodies. He'd seen the insides of hundreds of monkeys—and thousands of men, women, and children. Despite decades of practice, doing a transplant on nonhuman primates remained far more alien and unfamiliar. In the human body, White was at home. He could trace the spinal and cranial nerves with his eyes closed. White went over his notes one last time. He didn't need a new drug, not really. He didn't even need new equipment. Maintaining blood flow would be key, and monitoring the brain activity, too, but they did that now for most surgeries. What they would need, however, was fail-safe tech. He and Albin had developed it; the blood perfusion machine functioned almost like a mechanical heart and lung. It could propel and pump the blood as well as provide oxygen to both the body recipient and the transplant head during the critical middle steps.[41] If anything were to go wrong in the body transfer, the machine could do the heavy lifting so the brain would not be endangered. White went to the lab to examine the equipment, ticking off the items still necessary to purchase or duplicate. Then he returned to the dissection room. A call had come in, and he was in luck: two fresh bodies had just arrived. It was time for a trial run.

One lifeless cadaver lay upon White's surgery table. The newly dead look very like the sleeping living, except for the eyes peering up, unblinking. White touched the neck to draw a fine line all around its circumference, then pushed two metal hangers over the head, fastening them in place with screws into the head itself. Just out of view, on an identical operating table, was his "brain-dead" second cadaver. For the real surgery, two teams of surgeons, assistants, nurses, and anesthesiologists would wait in vibrating tension for scalpels to flash. White still needed his team for this, but they worked without quite the same angst—after all, the "patients" were in no danger of expiring.

White separated four of the six leads, the critical veins running under the skin, and connected them via coiled tubes to vessels in the "brain-dead" victim's torso. Were the hearts pumping, blood from both bodies would begin, now, to stream into the head of the first patient. White then carefully cut and sutured vessels until all relevant blood supply lines ran from the body to its new head. Another hour, and he had the cranium refastened to the "brain-dead" body, bolted in place to the vertebrae with screws and sutured, all the coiled tubes removed.[42] White checked the clock; the team had performed the surgery in good time. It had been a successful human version of the cephalic transplant—even if the "patients" were both expired.

Call it a head transplant or a body transplant; White had used both descriptors. But he insisted that the surgery planned for Vetovitz would *not* be an "experiment." You experimented on animals and on cadavers; a *clinical surgery* only went ahead when you had perfected it. White had spent almost thirty years refining even the smallest details. The head/body transplant had ceased to be an experiment in White's mind.[43] It was just a surgery yet to be performed.

## YOUR BIONIC FUTURE

"Next," White said, ushering aside the elderly woman with the numb fingers to make way for another client. A small crowd surrounded White at his "McDonald's office" near the clinic—a space where he could meet patients and give some free advice. It had started innocently enough;

he would be recognized, and then someone would ask his opinion on a medical complaint, and soon he found himself there regularly. A man in a dirty shirt shook White's hand. "Just wanted to say thanks," he said, smiling over stump teeth. "The headache is gone."[44] White nodded. That had been an easy one: change your brand of beer.

He'd be looking for a new McDonald's, out in Geneva, once his retirement was official. He could still be invited to conferences and boards after his retirement; he could even perform surgeries, so long as a hospital provided equipment and space. But there was something about being the only doctor—the single voice of reason and authority—that appealed in his work with the public. He enjoyed the feeling of rubbing elbows with life, especially in a space where no one had pretensions or expectations. Best of all, it was a good place to write. The lull of background noise (now largely missing at home) somehow jogged the brain cells. And White *needed* to write. His retirement festivities were approaching, followed by the enormous task of relocating an hour away, and he had a deadline to meet for *Scientific American*. It offered his best chance yet at publicizing the White Surgery, and would be his first time sharing the perfected protocol. The article would appear in late 1999, in the final months of the final year before the new millennium—when the twentieth century had become a "corpse outleant," as Thomas Hardy would say.* White was ready.

"Television and slot machines notwithstanding," wrote *Scientific American* editors Glenn Zorpette and Carol Ezzell in the opening of the issue, "the point of technology is to extend what we can do with

*The land's sharp features seemed to be
The Century's corpse outleant,
His crypt the cloudy canopy,
The wind his death-lament.
       —Thomas Hardy, "The Darkling Thrush," composed on December 31, 1899

our bodies, our senses, and most of all, our minds."[45] Calling the issue "Your Bionic Future," they referred to the dawn of a portable electronics age (though the iPhone was still eight years away), new discoveries in genetic codes and DNA, and something broadly described as "bionics." The term usually refers to cybernetic concepts—replacing human parts with techno-hardware—but for Zorpette and Ezzell, it also meant the "merger of the biological with the microelectronic" to transform human lives.[46] Within the next decade, they explained, we would see cloned humans, artificial wombs, organs grown from stem cells, sensory-rich virtual reality, custom body scans for clothing, and genetic vaccines that would allow us to build muscle without going to the gym.[47] Despite certain ambitious claims, the tone of the issue remains relatively restrained, focusing on things being researched and tested at the time. There were only three outliers, according to the editors, only three projects discussed in the magazine's pages that seemed too strange to be possible. The work of engineer Ray Kurzweil, for one, who argued that machines would attain emotions and consciousness. Dean Hamer was another of these fringe pioneers, for anticipating gene customization for babies that would reach even to personality. But the editors linger on a third seemingly outrageous contribution, an article titled "Head Transplants: Equipping Old Minds with New Bodies." *Surely, we won't see such a monster*, the editors conclude—but then again, the new millennium belonged to those willing to grasp the implications of a bionic future.

A tongue-in-cheek subheading—"Heads off to you"—appears above a photograph of an apparently alive and conscious head superimposed in a bell-shaped glass jar. "It is now possible," White begins, "to consider adapting the head-transplant technique to humans."[48] The essay describes the surgical protocol—the same protocol he had just practiced upon cadavers, the same he intended to use for Craig

Vetovitz—in detail. It read much the way his scientific publications on monkey head transplants did: authoritative but breezy and confident, accessible instead of overly academic. There was a notable change, however: White didn't call the subjects "preparations" anymore, the term he used to refer to monkeys. These were *patients*.

"Once the two patients were anesthetized," he wrote, using the past tense as though the surgery were already behind him, "the two teams" simultaneously made deep incisions around each patient's neck.[49] Bit by bit, they separated tissue and muscle to reach the carotid arteries, jugular veins, and spine.[50] At nearly five times the size of a monkey's, the human vascular system would be easy to locate, White explained, and far easier to work with. Bone would be excised from each patient's neck to expose the spinal cord and—just as with the macaques—each would be cleanly severed. He once more described the head removal, what he called the "critical maneuver," for everything after would be but the sewing up of veins and arteries, fastening together spinal columns and closing the skin.[51] There would be notable departures from the original surgery, of course; the second patient's head would no doubt be reverently removed. (For burial, perhaps?) And the now-useless body of the surviving head . . . well, it must surely go somewhere, too. White doesn't pause to speculate on the practice of burying one's "old" body once housed in a new one.

"My colleagues and I have already taken the first steps toward human head transplantation," White concluded, his words now flanked by an image of a head in his stabilizing C-clamp, which looked every bit like a neck-bolted Frankenstein's monster.[52] He enumerates the pumps for lowering body temperature to 10 degrees Celsius, his further development of cooling methods to slow metabolic rate. He also mentions the drugs necessary for preventing the body from rejecting its new head by suppressing immune response. More interesting, in retrospect, is what White does not say. He leaves out Craig Vetovitz's name, though he makes mention of a prospective patient facing possible organ failure. He also leaves out the name, still protected by anonymity, of the brain-dead patient White had chosen to be the body donor. We do know from Vetovitz, thanks to an episode of the Fox news program *A Current Affair*, that the male donor body was in excellent condition and the brain completely silent. We don't know more than this, nor what steps White had taken to get permission from the donor's family.

White's essay chooses to end with something more esoteric. Transplanting a human head was not only about scientific discovery; it was about preserving and extending life itself—a kind of immortality granted by trading up from a broken body. The real question wasn't how will we achieve this, White insisted, but rather "how well will society accept the concept that human brain transplantation involved transplanting the mind and spirit . . . the physical repository of the soul?"[53] Head transplant might save Craig Vetovitz's life, but it would do much, much more. It would (White was convinced) prove the location—and imply the existence—of the human soul . . . which may very possibly have been his principal goal all along.

Transplant surgery had always been about more than flesh and blood. Joseph Murray called transplant work a "surgery of the soul"; it gave him purpose and meaning. White meant to perform surgery *on* the soul. His own philosophy, his own speculation about where matter meets the immaterial, was but smoke in the wind without proof. A mind waking in a new body, eyes open and senses alert, though in a separate skin: this would be incontrovertible evidence that personhood lived in the brain, and that a four-dimensional soul could be transplanted in the confines of a three-dimensional head. "These are the questions," White concluded, "as we go in reality where Mary Wollstonecraft Shelley went only in fiction."[54]

. . .

The article hit press in late fall 1999. Within days, headlines across the world sizzled with anticipation. "Surgeon Plans Head Transplant!" announced the London *Times*.[55] Jonathan Leake, the article's author, claimed that the surgery would benefit "mortally ill tycoons" at the hefty cost of £800,000 per head. The most shocking aspect of the news story, however, wasn't the price tag; it was that the papers took for granted that the question was not *if* but *when*. A syndicated article in the *Taiwan News* and the *South China Morning Post* claimed that White, "the world's top brain surgeon," would be removing Craig Vetovitz's head at the Romadonaff Neurosurgery Institute in Ukraine—because, the article adds alarmingly, "the institute needs cash and the Ukraine's law on human organ transplant is lax." The piece went on to report that the $4 million bill would be picked up by the NIH and the Christopher & Dana Reeve Foundation.[56] There were, however, significant discrepancies between and among the articles. Some sources suggested that the surgery would take place in a Russian university and would cost $5 million; others said the Neuroscience Research Center of Kiev had first dibs. Just weeks later, a piece on White's proposed surgery (by then taken as imminent) appeared in the UK journal *Ethical Record* under the title "What Are the Prospects for Body Transplants?" Listing Craig Vetovitz alongside more famous names like Stephen Hawking and Christopher Reeve, the article doesn't just defend White's work as ethically sound, it suggests that paralytics deserved a healthy and longer life—paralysis and all. The author concluded, "*Mens sana in corpore sano*" (healthy minds in healthy bodies).[57] It might be surprising to find an ethics journal in such enthusiastic support of so disturbing a surgery—but not when the author was Harold Hillman, the same British neurobiologist who had traveled to Moscow to meet Demikhov and who was himself working on what he called "brain glue" in an attempt to stimulate regrowth of the spinal cord and cure paralysis.

Perhaps the new millennium fanned grand hopes, or perhaps the *Scientific American* article had at last hit the right chord; either way, a notable shift had occurred. Just a few years earlier, bioethicist Arthur Caplan had accused White's work of having a terminal "yuck factor" and complained that it "cheapened" life. Fellow neuroscientist Naomi Kleitman (a liaison for the Miami Project to Cure Paralysis) called it a "fantasy," and claimed that no one, not even her most disabled patients, would want such a surgery.[58] Now international newspapers weren't just chasing White, they were interviewing Vetovitz, too. "Everyone has to die sometime," Vetovitz told a Swedish paper.[59] He wasn't afraid to die for a cause. And White—despite his relocation to Geneva-on-the-Lake—now had a heavy speaking schedule booked around the two days a week he still spent at Metro, and had been featured in two documentaries. The spotlight had returned, and the Doctor Was In.

"I've named it the White Operation," he told *Wired* magazine in January 2000. He sensed a sea change. As the clocks and computers ticked over to the new millennium, no crash or technological disaster had occurred. Those who had stockpiled water, rations, ammunition, or even gold sheepishly went about dispersing their wares and clearing out their makeshift basement bunkers. Grander things were afoot. The first crew to live on the International Space Station arrived in space— US astronauts and Russian cosmonauts together, as a team. Scientists completed the first draft of the human genome, and White published a historical overview of brain transplant experiments in the journal *Neurological Research*. It would be, it *must* be, a century of the brain, he wrote. The question remained whether the United States would lead or be eclipsed by its rivals.

And yet, it was not to be. Vetovitz would complain bitterly to *A Current Affair* that "the government stepped in and put an end to the operation."[60] No hard evidence of that accusation has since come to light, but even before the end of 2000, it became clear that the surgery would not proceed in the United States. White had mentioned the Reeve Foundation in one of his interviews that year, but no funds had, in fact, been promised, and NIH grants were difficult to obtain for any research, much less the risky (and fringe) work of head transplants. News reports that the surgery had already been scheduled in Russia or the Ukraine were embellished, but the former Soviet Union did offer the best options for proceeding. "If we do this in Kiev," White said in August that year, "I think I can get the cost to two million."[61] Ukrainian institutions were, as White liked to describe them, "very unbureaucratic" when it came to surgery. Unlike the years of waiting for review board approvals in the United States, and extensive hours of training, White would only need three to four weeks to train a surgery team (possibly because the requirements for certification were less stringent), and about the same amount of time to "clear up the formalities with authorities."[62] White had been elected to membership in both the Russian and Ukrainian academies of medical sciences; he'd performed surgeries there, too, even on that first visit to Moscow in 1966. And at the very least, a transplant body would be easy enough to find.[63] White told *Wired* that he'd received letters of invitation from Moscow, Leningrad, and Kiev. "They all want me," he said.[64] But he would not be asked to perform another surgery at Cleveland Metropolitan General Hospital. He had officially (and with some bitterness) retired.

## FROM RUSSIA WITH LOVE

The work of a lifetime never fits in a single room. White's office boxes and all their hidden treasures had migrated to three separate locations.

He'd been assigned an "emeritus" office at Metro, a room he shared with a few other retired faculty who couldn't quite let go of the hospital and all that it meant. His home office in Shaker Heights, full to the brim already, took a few odds and ends, and the rest followed him to Geneva-on-the-Lake. The lake house had a more modern feel to it, right down to the Formica desk and bank of sliding windows that overlooked the shore. The walls had been freshly hung with his awards, black-and-white photos of the first isolation surgeries, and pictures of the pope. Two portraits he regarded as worthy of special consideration. The first was of Harvey Cushing, often considered the father of neurosurgery. The second belonged to a man White had met: Dr. Vladimir Negovsky, the Soviet father of "reanimatology" (resuscitation) and the uses of hypothermia, fields of study that made him the inheritor of Sergei Brukhonenko's *Experiments in the Revival of Organisms*.

White had made return trips to Russia. He had even been back to the Institute of the Brain with a CBS television crew in 1992. At last, they let White into the mythic Room 19, where the accumulated brains of prominent leaders were suspended in formaldehyde—even Lenin's was there.[65] Claimed to be missing for years, Lenin's brain had, in fact, been sliced into an astonishing 30,000 pieces. Paper thin, carefully preserved, and nearly transparent, the slides were all that remained of the mind behind the revolution. "I held in my hand a section of the brain of a man who was responsible for murdering millions of people and who had created a form of Communist government that still exists in many countries all over the world," White told the camera crew. It was an honor he'd been waiting three decades for, a mark of regard and trust that he appreciated—but he was also only too glad to leave.[66] It was one thing to make a museum of pathology, a reminder of successes and failures and the endless pursuit of better neurological care. It was another to be in the presence, even fleetingly, of Vladimir Lenin and all the history that went with him. But perhaps the most surprising thing about White's trip wasn't the wonders he witnessed, but the seemingly everyday objects that took on mythic proportions for the Russians he met. One colleague spirited White away that day to show him the Institute of the Brain's prized possession: an early Apple computer. Just one.[67] And things had not improved very much in the new millennium.

By 2000, Russia was in a period of transition. Boris Yeltsin had control, but the effects of his government's instability were deeply apparent.[68] Street crime had escalated, especially pickpocketing and cash grabs at busy markets. The country's currency had collapsed, too, and people struggled to eke out a living. It didn't feel like freedom; it felt a lot more like poverty. Even the cabdrivers complained about the misery inflicted upon them by the "West," and by Americans specifically (though no one could say exactly how).[69] The prime minister, Vladimir Putin, had his eye on the presidency, eager to establish some order. He'd get his wish on May 7, riding a wave of nostalgia for more stable Soviet times, and would immediately restore the Soviet national anthem from 1944.

White might have had plenty of invitations from colleagues in Russia and Ukraine to honor their institutions with his revolutionary surgery, but it came down to cost, cost, cost. Even at its least expensive, the full-body transplant required significant sums. Yes, the Iron Curtain had lifted, but hospitals were strapped for cash—and labs and medical techniques remained some ten or fifteen years behind technologically. If White wanted to perform the transplant surgery in the former USSR, he would have to supply the funds himself.

The irony was that White could have done the surgery in 1975. He was told that identical twin brothers had been arrested, convicted, and sentenced to death in Kiev. White had been invited to try on humans what he had done on monkeys, using the brothers as his subjects; the Kiev labs were at his disposal. Surely *these* were the perfect patients. Should the surgery fail, they would have died under anesthetic, perhaps less painfully than by execution.[70] Should it succeed, White could have proven the White Principle: that the human soul was mobile, that it could be moved, and that a body transplant could save the life of a mind trapped in a dying body. But that wasn't how it worked. A surgeon of any ethics would never operate on patients against their will—especially not on (possibly political) prisoners. And White had needed all the years that followed to create a surgery protocol he felt would be safe enough for a clinical trial. PETA had called him Dr. Frankenstein, yes, but they had been wrong about one thing: White did care about the means as well as the end. Scientific progress wasn't everything. In the sea of ethics and morality, White once said, "there are no navigation maps." The only lodestone is a man's conscience.[71]

In Russia, White would no doubt have found support at any of the institutions he mentioned as candidates, but not funding. ("I looked in the mail today," he joked to one reporter, and strangely enough "didn't see a check for $2 million.")[72] In the United States, there was certainly money to be had, but White's surgery would get no support. By the following September, not quite two years into White's retirement, the Twin Towers would come down. The heady optimism of a new millennium had turned to the dread of terrorism and the threat of war in the Middle East. Perhaps it was this sudden shift in focus, or perhaps the age of racing other nations for scientific prowess had simply come to an abrupt end. Either way, the monkey transplants, once considered cutting-edge research, were increasingly cast as macabre, fringe science. His skeptics' chief complaint didn't concern brain death, or even White's animal experimentation. It had to do with the severed spine.

White had always accepted that his surgery's chief limitation would be a paralyzed patient. It's one reason he focused so much on figures who were already paralyzed; to them, the surgery was a means of extending the life they had, not getting a better one. White did hold out hope that, one day, science might solve that problem, too—but his principal aim had always been the proof of concept. After all, the first heart transplants did not improve the recipients' lives, and even possibly shortened them. Yet without those first surgeries, the extensive practice of the truly lifesaving heart transplants we have today would never have become a reality. To White, his innovation was worthy in much the same way; to his critics, however, it was a step too far. No one wanted to support such a drastic surgical intervention unless the results led to the rehabilitation of the patient, not merely a continuation of their quadriplegia.

In an interview with CBS, Dr. Jerry Silver, a neurologist at White's own Case Western Reserve University, decried White's work. Silver had been in the lab in 1970 when White's monkey awoke, completely paralyzed. "It was just awful," he recounted. "I don't think it should ever be done again." Since reattaching the human spinal cord was "pure and utter fantasy," performing a head transplant would render a patient forever paralyzed; for Silver, even if the patient were paralyzed to begin with, that kind of experimental surgery should simply "never happen."[73] Dr. Steven Rose, director of brain research at the Open University in the UK, agreed. He attacked White in a 2001 interview with BBC News, calling his work "entirely misleading, technically irrelevant, and apart from anything else, a grotesque breach of any ethical consideration."[74] White's rebuttal, quoted in the same article, that "people are dying today who, if they had body transplants, in the spinal injury community would remain alive," did not move his opponents.[75] From St Bartholemew's Hospital in London, Dr. Peter Hamlyn called White's research "cruel" and irrelevant, and men like Vetovitz "cranks" seeking attention.[75] White was more hurt by the attacks upon his would-be patient than those on himself. How could a doctor direct such words to a man whose body was failing him, and who wanted life to go on, however limited that life might be?

Sometime success breeds its own discontents. The first heart transplant patient had lived only a few scant weeks; those who followed, mere months. They had nonetheless been hailed as proof that transplants saved lives. In the decades that followed, survival rates bloomed, but the criteria for recipients contracted. Vetovitz had been denied a kidney transplant because a disabled body was not thought of as a "good candidate." For better or worse, surgical protocols had come to be measured by medical professionals' opinions on what constituted a life well lived. Vetovitz was living proof. He still looked for new possibilities, still fought for stem cell research. Where was America's enthusiasm for experimentation, its passion for attempting what had never before been done? It seemed the obstacle facing the quadriplegic was the same afflicting the White Surgery: *paralysis*.

But what if you *could* reknit that bundles of nerves and unblock the superhighway of information between brain to body? What might happen if a cure could be found, medically or technologically, that restored and reanimated the paralyzed body? Would White's surgery at last be allowed to proceed? The answer lingered on the near horizon of that so-called "bionic future." It would be called *BrainGate*.

# Chapter 9

# WHAT IF WE DON'T NEED THE SPINAL CORD?

*On January 24, 2000, investment company Nuveen released an ad created for* Super Bowl XXXIV. In the minute-long spot, Christopher Reeve, the *Superman* actor paralyzed in 1995, stands up from his chair and walks. The ad caused a firestorm. CGI technology, now so familiar, was still incredibly new. The imagery looked *real*, and viewers flooded the phone lines. Where had Reeve gone to receive the cure, and could they get it, too? Nuveen, an investment firm, bought the ad space for $4 million, claiming that it wanted to inspire investors to give to charities like Reeve's (instead of buying "bigger boats").[1] The company and ABC (which aired the Super Bowl that year) were accused of being grossly misleading, but Reeve insisted the scene portrayed in the ad was "something that can actually happen." Reeve would not live to see the day, but his words were remarkably prescient. Just two years later, Cyberkinetics Neurotechnology Systems Inc., a Brown University medical device start-up, sought permission to launch pilot clinical trials of a first-generation *neural interface system*. They wanted to implant a device inside the human brain that would send signals directly to muscles, bypassing severed spinal nerves. Research teams at Brown, Massachusetts General Hospital, Stanford University, Providence VA Medical Center, and Dr. White's own Case Western Reserve University had all begun to ask a provocative question: What if we don't need the spinal cord? What if a patient could move just by thinking?

## ENTER BRAINGATE

Dr. John Donoghue, head of the neuroscience department at Brown, began studying how the brain translates thought into action in the 1980s—and later studied how to translate these electronic impulses into the (likewise electrical) language of computers and mechanical commands.[2] Theoretically, his research offered the first opportunity to allow the brain to jump the spinal cord and communicate directly with the limbs. Brown didn't have the resources necessary to create the technology that might enable this; but the University of Utah had been developing advanced neuro-sensor chips, which would be able to measure and transmit neural activity as electrical impulse.* Donoghue teamed up with researchers there and filed paperwork for laboratory animals to begin testing their products. Shortly after, he received his first rhesus macaque.[3]

Donoghue's experimental macaque would be taught to perform tasks, a bit like White's PhD monkeys. As a new-millennium primate, it was trained on digital video games instead of analog machines, learning to use a joystick to move a cursor for a treat reward. Donoghue's surgical team then anesthetized the monkey and implanted an electronic

---

*Under normal circumstances, the brain is doing this all the time: transmitting information via electrical signals to move parts of the body.

chip deep into its brain.[4] Team members hooked up the monkey's neural chip directly to a computer. To get the reward, the monkey had to move the cursor once again—but without using a joystick at all. Instead, it had to *think* about the joystick movement; in so doing, electrical impulses from the monkey's own brain moved the cursor on the computer screen. In almost miraculous fashion, a thought had been electrically translated into action without the aid of the spinal cord for the very first time.

Donoghue chose *Nature* to publish the article announcing his success, just as White had decades before. "Instant Neural Control," as the piece was called, claimed the new technology could be used by paralyzed patients—not to control their own limbs (or not yet) but to interact with the world around them merely by thinking.[5] It caused a sensation, and generated a flurry of coverage in other publications, like *Science*'s "Monkey See, Cursor Do," which claimed "The animals could 'think' the cursor onto the target just as quickly as they could move it there by hand."[6] But Donoghue still didn't know *what* the monkeys were thinking; they couldn't speak to him, couldn't explain what the sensation was like. For that, he would need to use the device on humans. He cofounded Cyberkinetics Neurotechnology Systems Inc. with his Brown colleagues Mijail Serruya and Gerhard Friehs, professors of neurology and neurosurgery, respectively, and Nicho Hatsopoulos, chairman of computational neuroscience at the University of Chicago. Together, they set about getting the device financed and FDA-approved for clinical trials.

In 2004, hospitals in Rhode Island, Massachusetts, and Illinois were approved as sites for the pilot trial. Four participants with tetraplegia agreed to enroll.[7] The surgeries proceeded without complications, but unfortunately, the trial proved cumbersome and time-consuming, requiring two months of lessons and then hours of practice to move the cursor—and this in the context of the patients' everyday lives. Cyberkinetics would spend two more years refining the neural interface system. Then, surgeons implanted the sensor into the brain of a twenty-five-year-old Rhode Island resident, Matthew Nagle, a onetime high school football star who'd become paralyzed after being stabbed in the neck at a Fourth of July celebration three years before. They hooked up his brain to a prosthetic arm. Soon, he could open and close the hand by just thinking of the action. Then, he lifted the arm straight into the air. "Holy shit!" he exclaimed; he hadn't moved his own arms and legs in years, but now he had waved to the surgeons *using only his mind.*[8]

For Donoghue, the study's most important finding wasn't that humans could do as monkeys could. Researchers worried that neural pathways might atrophy, or be rerouted. But the signals in Nagle's brain that used to control his arm movements were still functional, even years after his injury. It proved that the thoughts that speak to our arms, to our fingers and toes, that wrinkle a nose or raise an eyebrow, remain active even when sensory input has been denied for long periods of time. To Donoghue, this meant that future implants wouldn't just move robotic limbs; they would move the patient's *own.* It meant that curing paralysis might not rely on fixing the spinal cord. You didn't need to fix what you could bypass.[9]

Nagle's BrainGate Neural Interface System implant was about the size of a baby aspirin. One hundred thin, hairlike electrodes protruded from one side. The device rested just above a region in the brain known to control motor activity. For Nagle, the chip was designed to work only one way: he would send out thoughts, which became electrical signals, which translated into external motion. With other models, however, the process had feedback. Donoghue suggested that "deep brain electrodes" slipped up to four inches into the brain could be used to alleviate chronic pain or might have implications for other diseases, such as Parkinson's, epilepsy, and depression.[10] But David Ewing Duncan, a journalist and author of *Experimental Man*, wrote a responding article for *SFGate* charging that if the brain can be fed impulses, might that evolve into mind control? Or might devices like Nagle's allow fighter pilots to fly jets and fire missiles with only their thoughts—a strange return to the bizarre telekinetic experiments of Soviet Russia? Donoghue admitted that a performance artist had hooked up electrical impulses to his stomach to control a third arm with ten fingers, activating the motor cells by using his stomach muscles.[11] Still, Nagle shrugged off any possible negative consequences, assured that God was using him to show the world what the future could be like. "I have no regrets," he said. "I hope this brings hope to other people."[12]

It certainly did—and not just to those with paralysis. One neurosurgeon in particular had been following Donoghue's research very, very keenly.

Dr. White ordered coffee and settled into his preferred table at the McDonald's in Geneva, Ohio. It wasn't much to look at, just the usual décor of a roadside stop off a busy freeway. White had asked for a special parking spot—nothing *too* grand, but wouldn't it be nice to have a free space painted with the words "DR. WHITE"? The manager thought he'd been joking about using the restaurant as his office. When he realized the elderly fellow in the ball cap and bifocals actually meant what he said, he agreed on a compromise. White's table remained permanently reserved, complete with an official-looking nameplate. Connie, who owned the nearby Sunrise Café, put his name on a special chair.

At seventy-four, White had been retired for five years, but retirement didn't stop his brain from whirring, didn't stop his excitement over every new possibility in the wide world of neuroscientific research. There was still so much he could do—he wanted to stay involved, integral, important. He took up a post as consultant for Medical Mutual health insurance, a position as visiting professor at St. George's University School of Medicine in Grenada, and additional work as a member of the Pontifical Academy of Sciences, giving papers and being part of discussions about the Church's stance on stem cells and when life *began*. He visited Metro regularly, sometimes spending the night in the house he and Patricia still owned in Shaker Heights, and served as an expert reviewer and occasional editor for medical papers and journals. He also, more humbly, wrote a regular column in the local *News-Herald*. Sometimes it offered the only place for his more personal voice, his attempts to stay ahead of the times and, perhaps, to stay relevant.

So when news of BrainGate appeared, crackling with all the excitement of science fiction, he sat down at his McDonald's desk to write about it. "What we are all witnessing is a true revolution in health care," White wrote. "With future advances in these technologies many incurable neurological and psychiatric diseases will become treatable, establishing a new health specialty of 'brain engineering.'"[13] If professional jealousy had any hand in the writing, it doesn't show. White talked instead about opportunity and how wires might one day be used to leap connections between brain and body. Even so, the larger neuroscientific community remained skeptical. "It is a lot of hype, a lot of entertainment," complained Dr. Miguel Nicolelis, an associate professor of neurobiology at Duke University, in an echo of charges leveled against White's own groundbreaking work.[14] They were putting wires in the brain, sending and receiving messages; even if mind control wasn't really a threat, they still needed regulations—and to keep maverick science and patient risk at bay.

With this, White seemed to agree. "My youngest daughter-in-law asked me the other day if science could now create zombies, [and] I initially thought the question was silly," he wrote.[15] But perhaps it wasn't so far-fetched. He had been reviewing the experimental work on brain stimulation, particularly work on animals where the control and behavioral centers had been aroused or compromised. White knew of studies where brain stimulation altered animal character and response: a bull no longer wanted to charge, a rat became obsessed with giving itself sensations of pleasure. (The rat sadly pleasured itself to death.) He never called Donoghue's work sensationalist or macabre, but he didn't spare his thoughts on the possible scenarios where things might go wrong. It remained a *brain surgery*, after all, with all the potential problems that went along with that. "In the short run," he wrote, "it could fail by causing hemorrhage in the brain, if the electrode placement is inappropriate. In the long run, there might be infection or battery and equipment failure."[16] The brain was not a playground. But BrainGate had answers for that, too.[17]

As an operation for installing the electrodes began, the surgery team would fasten a special device called a stereotactic helmet to the patient's head to immobilize it. A clear plastic bubble with protrusions at the top and sides, the helmet looked like some imagined astronaut headgear from early sci-fi movies. Within the hemisphere, monitors for magnetic resonance imaging (MRI) swept across the patient's head, using high-frequency radio waves to provide images from which the surgeons could construct a brain map.[18] The neurosurgeons no longer operated blind; for BrainGate surgeries, they could see exactly where to place an electrode to stimulate some part of the brain. Only a tiny incision needed to be made in the scalp, a small hole drilled in the skull, and then the electrodes slowly entered the interior. The patient, up till that point, remained awake. They needed him to. His responses helped the surgeons coordinate the data from within the helmet with the MRI scan views. Every brain retains its little mysteries, so they needed patient cooperation to be sure stimulation occurred in exactly the right place—*Do you feel this in your hand? In your toes?* Only when they were satisfied that patient responses put them in the right place for stimulation would the patient be put under, leaving the neurosurgeon to "tunnel under the tissues," as White put it, of the head, neck, and chest.[19] A stimulating unit would be mounted under the skin of the chest, a bit like a pacemaker, boosting signals that passed through, and wires would be connected from those brain electrodes to the corresponding muscles. Once awake, and trained to its use, the patient would be able to stimulate himself. *What if* such a device could allow someone to walk again? Could enough electrodes be placed, with enough specificity, to allow transmission all the way to the arms and legs? And if so . . . would the world be prepared, once and for all, for the White Surgery?

White could clearly see the benefits of all those electrical gadgets potentially solving the severing of the spinal cord. If BrainGate's system really and truly worked, his meticulous protocol might, at last, be put to the clinical test. But if so, it would very likely not be White who performed the surgery. On his sojourns to the Metro office, he sometimes encountered an emergency team rushing to prep for brain surgery. He felt it like a surge, muscle memory encouraging him to jump from his chair and scrub in. He loved it. He went so far as to call it his one real drug. But White hadn't operated in five years. He had been busy doing other things.

## YOU HAVE BEEN X-FILED

In early September 2007, White put on his lab coat, waiting quietly in the emeritus surgeons' office at Metro. He expected a guest, and meeting *here* lent him a sense of authority.

His daughter Patty had set up the meeting. There had been a few recently—including one with a young filmmaker who'd done a documentary on the head transplant surgery for *Vice*. Aware of the usual financial restrictions, Patty had offered this newest interviewer the standard options: she knew the cheapest hotels to stay at, the best restaurants for getting a hearty but inexpensive meal, and did he need to be picked up from the airport? No, said the man's personal assistant; he will be flying in by private jet. Dr. White's visitor would be Frank Spotnitz, executive producer of *The X-Files*.

Spotnitz had begun as a writer for the popular television series, responsible for writing or cowriting forty episodes before ultimately producing the show's first companion feature film. He had just begun work on the film's sequel, *I Want to Believe*, when he ran into a bit of a snag. As part of the plot, Spotnitz intended to have one character perform a head transplant on his lover, and he wanted to stay as close to "real" science as possible. He asked his research assistant to poke around in medical history, and only a short while later, the assistant called him in breathless excitement: *It's not fiction*, he explained. Someone—a surgeon in Cleveland—had *actually done it*. Spotnitz wanted to meet the man. Partly, of course, as research. But also out of legitimate curiosity. What sort of person took the heads off monkeys? "It's always very exciting to me," Spotnitz later explained, "when I come up with a story plucked out of thin air, out of my imagination, and it has a basis in reality."[20] To think that it had truly occurred struck him with horror and fascination in equal measure.

The meeting was private; there would be no cameras, no published article to record the event—only the deep impressions made on a science fiction filmmaker. Spotnitz found himself by turns impressed, touched, and uncomfortable with the man before him. Soft-spoken, polite, even gentle, "a lovely, grandfatherly man" who nevertheless spoke about cutting through monkeys' spinal cords with cool detachment . . .[21] "I've hit a dead end," White admitted to Spotnitz;

the severed spinal cord could not be reattached, and no one would risk the surgery without a solution to the paralysis that resulted. Or rather, no one would risk it *unless* new research bypassing the spinal cord were to prove successful. Spotnitz asked him about the monkeys: Why so many monkeys? Wasn't it horrible? White remained serene. He had no qualms whatsoever; he never had. It was the emotional detachment, finally, that made the meeting so memorable to Spotnitz. "What stayed with me," he recalled years later, during work on the Prime Video series *The Man in the High Castle*, "was my impression of *the man*, supremely untroubled by the implications of his work."[22]

For Spotnitz, the value of science fiction lay in its ability to help us see those very implications more clearly. "We go into research with faith that we're heading in the right direction," Spotnitz suggested. "It's only after technology has lunged forward that we understand what we have done."[23] In fiction, the ethics have a face, a plot, a narrative through line. We care about it; we see ourselves in it. Fiction offers a space where human questions can be explored in safety: Will we accommodate ourselves to these new realities? Will we allow them, even in the face of their potential consequences? This is the value of fiction, according to Spotnitz: not that we see such fantasies as models, but that we see them as cautionary tales. The inventions of the Industrial Revolution brought with them the accidents of that future, and we often cannot know the consequences until we arrive. All the same, we must take care not to invent the train crash *before* the train . . . And yet, in meeting Dr. White, Spotnitz had stumbled into the darkest reaches of his own imagination and found what lurked there to be *real*.[24] Perhaps, he suggested, this was the collective unconscious at work, the idea that all humankind is connected by ancient and invisible threads to ancestral memory and primal fear. *Perhaps.*

*The X-Files: I Want to Believe* premiered on July 25, 2008, and grossed

$4 million on opening day. The film made over $68 million by the end of its international run. Though critics complained of its "body parts, gruesomeness, gloom and doom,"[25] Roger Ebert gave the movie three-and-a-half out of four stars. "It's not simply about good and evil," he wrote, "but about choices," making it a good horror thriller.[26] The concept of a head transplant had become the stuff of monster movies once again. White was credited as a medical consultant on the film, but the White Surgery was no longer proper science; it had reverted to the stuff of science fiction. And while White claimed to be proud of his pop culture influence, a neurosurgeon could not build his legacy upon *The X-Files*.

## WHEN THE DOCTOR IS THE PATIENT

The room was unfamiliar. Dimmed fluorescent lights revealed sterile walls, a buff-colored curtain pulled aside with metal clips, and a distant monitor. Indistinct noises filtered through from one side; the sound of rubber soles on worn linoleum. Dr. White blinked his eyes to clear his bleary vision. Gone were the windows facing Lake Erie; instead, the tops of buildings stretched across a cold November skyline. *We've come to show you the MRI scans,* a Dr. Columbi explained. White knew the name; Columbi had been his student. He'd asked for him and Dr. Selman (another former pupil) specifically, before his thinking grew confused. *You've been in an accident,* they told him, holding up images of a brain. For a moment, it might have been years earlier, when they were students and he the knowing professor showing them scans. But the brain belonged to Dr. White this time, and a hazy whiteness between skull and gray matter told him everything he needed to know: he had suffered a subdural hematoma.[27] A brain bleed.

It was early November, just months after the *X-Files* premiere.

White had gone for groceries in his charcoal-colored Grand Am. The trip home wasn't a long one; he'd done it once a week for ages, the same market, the same road, the same parking lot. White had nosed the sedan onto Route 534 to the tinny plinking of his turn signal; then everything went *bang*. He didn't have the right of way, and had been hit by an oncoming car. The undercarriage absorbed the shock, yet even the slightest collision jars the body with a force that seems greater than the velocity should make possible. Unprepared, White rocked forward in his seat, forehead thumping soundly on the driver's-side door. The couple driving the other car called the police, and someone phoned White's son Michael, who lived nearby. *Just a fender bender*, White explained. He had a cut on his scalp and the woman in the other car had bumped her arm, but no one went to the hospital. Michael drove White home with a bad bruise forming. Patricia fussed over him, of course—she knew from years of being married to a neurosurgeon that slight bangs could do plenty of damage. White insisted he just needed a lie-down. By the next day, however, something seemed very wrong. His words were slurred and his mind was fuzzy. By day three, confused and shaken, White asked Michael to call University Hospital.[28]

A spinal surgeon as well as brain surgeon, Dr. Columbi had operated on White once before for a damaged disc. (Columbi had been on a ski vacation shortly before the operation, but had refused to step foot on the slopes; what if he got injured and couldn't operate on his mentor?)[29] White trusted him; he ought to, having taught him. To the untrained eye, the black-and-gray image Columbi held before him would reveal only the fuzzy outline of a skull and a great quantity of rippled nothingness between the outer wall and the inner ventricles. To White, it spoke of ruptured vessels and blood pooled into the soft tissue. White had effectively suffered a stroke. Subdural hematomas had killed countless of his patients; White had saved others only to have them make stuttering and incomplete recoveries. He wanted to rise, to get up from the bed—but his balance had deserted him. He could scarcely keep his head up. Columbi admitted him immediately to neurosurgical intensive care.

White hadn't wanted to retire. He hadn't wanted to give up the hospital. Now he suddenly worried he wouldn't be allowed out of it in time for Christmas. Who would play Santa for the students at the Saturday Scholars program for disadvantaged children at Lomond School—who would buy the presents on the teachers' curated list?[30] Would he have to relearn to walk? Had his mind been permanently affected? And what about *his work?*

Months later, White was still in rehab. "It reminded me of . . . the *Picture of Dorian Gray,*" he wrote in his *News-Herald* column. White imagined himself as Dorian, remaining "young, healthy, and with a good physical appearance compared to . . . my fellow patients in the physical and occupational classes," whose bodies betrayed their faults and flaws while he stayed morally and spiritually "ageless."[31] But back in his small, white room, looking into the bath mirror under unforgiving fluorescent light, White knew the truth. The face peering back had age spots; it was sunken and jowled and loose of skin. "It suddenly dawned on me that I really wasn't any different from the patients," White admitted, honest and raw though it was. *We are the same* "in our common desire to survive and return" to the world.[32]

White the humble. White the butcher. White the experimental surgeon with hundreds of articles and thousands of surgeries to his name, who had designed perfusion techniques and cephalic transplants, who had wanted to create the first true head/body transplant for a human being—this same Dr. White was only mortal. And whatever slim, hairsbreadth of hope had lingered on since his plucky announcement eight years before that the time for a head transplant was at long last nigh, White knew now that he would never perform another surgery.

While in rehab, as if in answer to his own failing health, White received word that new management at Metro planned to dismantle the Brain Research Lab. The floor had been vacant for eight years now, a little museum within the hospital. Without funding, his former group couldn't carry on with his research and had moved on to other things— and anyway, White had taken his monkey experiments pretty much as far as they could go. Metro needed the space. He could take what he wanted, they said. The rest would be thrown away. In fact, some files had already been destroyed, mere detritus from surgeries that would never be done again. No one, it seemed, had seen the point of a surgery that saved heads at the expense of a functional body.

By spring, White's own physical body had begun to degrade. He'd had several more health scares, including recurrent gastric bleeding that had meant at least one terrifying helicopter ride in the stormy dark. Even once home again, unable to drive, unable to walk unassisted, his health became increasingly fragile. His lab had already been disassembled, his carefully preserved boxes relocated to free corners of the Geneva house. Of all the things that had transpired, White took that news the hardest. He'd hoped his work might be preserved, even if only as a museum, in the hospital to which he'd given most of his life. Of course, some of his work *had* been preserved—or rather, *employed*. Around the country, neurosurgeons were treating spinal cord injuries, major ischemia, strokes, and head trauma using perfusion cooling.[33] All had been anchored in White's earlier experiments: in the isolation of the brain and, before that, in the perfusion of dogs and monkeys. That work would go on. Without acolytes to carry his full-body transplant protocol into the future, perfusion seemed to be the only thing left to White—the only achievement not yet forgotten, even if he feared that he himself might be.

Life, White had said, was the most important thing to preserve. But with his own life and career ebbing, White began to think far more seriously about preserving *legacy*. And so, in late January 2010, White sat down to write a letter. He needed help from an old friend.

"Dear Bob," wrote Joseph Murray in reply just days later. "Thanks for your carefully planned helpful letter about the Nobel Prize. . . . I am taking appropriate steps allowable under the current guidelines for nominations."[34] At White's request, Murray, as a former winner of the Nobel Prize himself, had agreed to nominate him to take his place among the distinguished names of scientific greats.

As one of that august crowd—men and women whose service to future generations had been recognized in physics, chemistry, medicine, literature, peace, and economics—White would attain a legacy held by fewer than one thousand people, only about two hundred of whom had hailed from the fields of physiology or medicine. One of them had been Demikhov's idol, Ivan Pavlov, another the French surgeon Alexis Carrel, the man who had so long ago swapped the legs of dogs (though without much success). Watson and Crick (of double-helix DNA fame) had made the grade in 1962 . . . and of course Joseph Murray himself, in 1990. In at least one way, it was still possible to live forever.

The Nobel Prize has its history in the life and fortune of Alfred Nobel. Born in Sweden and raised in Russia, the industrialist left the lion's share of his estate to the establishment of a monetary prize in 1895. The Nobel Prize for Physiology or Medicine belongs only to those who have made discoveries that have "changed the scientific paradigm and are of great benefit for mankind." Neither lifetime achievement or scientific leadership matter. The contribution must be a specific discovery, and it must have the promise of standing the test of ages. A select few may nominate candidates for the prize, principally past winners in the same category—that is, men like Joseph Murray.

"The history of this nomination actually begins at the Peter Bent Brigham Hospital," wrote Murray in the opening paragraphs of his proposal.[35] It was here, he went on to explain, that Dr. White worked with Francis Moore and with Murray himself, excited by the "investigative spirit" of Moore's laboratory. The young White, home from the war, still shocked at his good fortune in securing a place at Harvard, still formidable of physique, still wearing those black-rimmed glasses: this same White would go on to do remarkable work at the Mayo Clinic, where he developed the very first perfusion unit for his hemispherectomy surgeries, resulting in the complete circulatory arrest of the brain—an on-off switch, so to speak. Murray listed seven major accomplishments of White's life, beginning with the isolation of the primate brain and followed in order by brain perfusion (cooling till the metabolism nearly stops), the discovery of the protective effect of deep hypothermia, the long-term storage of cold brains, the treatment of spinal injuries using hypothermia, the transplantation of the brain into the neck of a dog, and the transplantation of the head itself onto another body. But though the last of these might have been the most forward-looking, Murray spent no time discussing it further. The single, significant work—the work for which Murray felt White deserved recognition as a Nobel laureate—had nothing to do with transplants, and everything to do with cooling technology.

White's "experimental work dealing with the effects of deep hypothermia on central nervous system tissue" Murray speaks of almost as though it were science fiction, calling it "impossible to believe." White had proven beyond doubt that a supercooled brain could be put almost in stasis—bloodless, without circulation, and seemingly "dead"—for long periods of time, only to be revived again with no ill effects. "Just contemplate what this means," Murray insisted: not only can the brain—with its delicate, sensitive, intricate, and necessary operations—*survive* temperatures seemingly at odds with life, it may be *protected* by them.[36] The great advancements of cardiovascular and neurosurgery had been made possible by putting the brain in circulatory arrest; it allowed for longer and more delicate operations. Successful operations on hard-to-reach tumors, even reconstructions to the aorta, owed their success to White's pioneering work. This above all else, Murray claimed, was White's defining achievement. He had learned to put a head on ice to preserve its function, and so, too, sustain the personality—the *self*—housed within. Wasn't that worthy of recognition?

Murray would not spend much time on White's other, less salubrious work. No part of the proposal would make even passing mention of the utility of head transplants for human beings. When Murray had asked White (before drafting his nomination) for a concise summary of his work in perfusion, he'd cautioned his colleague against his loquacious tendencies; *not one extra word* should be in the document—and no mention of a full-body transplant, either. "No need for you to be embarrassed," he'd told White. "I am happy to help."[37] He signed the message "your fellow lab jockey" and promised to do what he could to get the proposal before the committee. *But*, he warned, "our correspondence must be kept STRICTLY confidential."[38] Of course, strictly speaking, White shouldn't even *know* that he had been nominated. The names of nominees (and their nominators) were expected, by the rules of the Nobel committee, to remain sealed for fifty years, guaranteeing anonymity. That the members of the nominating committees did not themselves always abide by the rules might be taken as read.

White had slipped Murray an updated CV, too, writing over the old copy in pencil (with his unusual block capital letters and curlicues) and giving the mess to his daughter Patty to type. In the end, it ran for twelve full pages. He had earned a BS, an MD, and a PhD. He held four honorary degrees as well: two doctor of science degrees, one doctor of humane letters, and one doctor of arts and sciences. White had held thirteen different appointments in medicine, edited three major journals (*Surgical Neurology*, *Resuscitation*, and *Journal of Trauma*), and sat on several editorial boards. He belonged to fifty-eight societies in several countries, sat on numerous boards of trustees, and was the recipient of many, many awards and honors. White wanted very much to add one more, but for once, it was entirely out of his hands. He must sit—and wait.

## THE BRAIN-COMPUTER INTERFACE

*Sitting. Waiting.* Still early in 2010, but across the Atlantic in Zurich, Switzerland, surgeons delivered bad news to a young gymnast. Twenty-year-old college student David Mzee had done a flip off the trampoline and onto a foam pad. The cushioning should have broken his fall, but Mzee instead broke his neck. He would spend months in physical therapy, and though he regained the use of his upper body, his spinal nerves had been too damaged to allow him the use of his legs—particularly his left leg. He would spend his life in a wheelchair, like so many before him.[39]

Gertjan Oskan, an engineer from the Netherlands, was hit by a car the following year. Surgeons told him, on his twenty-eighth birthday, that he would be paralyzed for life. Some months later, Sebastian Tobler, a keen cyclist, badly damaged his spine in a mountain biking accident. Doctors explained that his spinal cord had gone "silent"; his legs would never work again.[40] In each of these three cases, the spinal cord damage could not be healed—bundles of nerves had been killed off from injury and swelling and a suicide domino effect, where the dying nerves sent signals that triggered the deaths of others nearby. In each case, the patients struggled to adapt to a life of new limitations . . . and in each case, they waited and watched and hoped for some break-through. Craig Vetovitz had described feeling helpless, and the frustra-tion of relying on those you wanted to protect and support. He'd been willing to do the impossible, to sign up for White's full-body transplant surgery to stay alive, having long ago given up the dream of regain-ing his mobility. But there would be a great difference between what was possible for Vetovitz, paralyzed in 1977, and what was possible for these three men, who became paralyzed in 2010 and 2011. Mzee, Oskan, and Tobler would all walk again. They would do it by skipping over their spinal cord damage and going "cyborg."

BrainGate had not been idle. By 2015, BrainGate researchers, led by David Borton at Brown, had performed a full proof-of-concept study. Like White before them, they would use rhesus macaques as test sub-jects. The team used a surgically induced spinal injury to render two monkeys paralyzed in one hind leg. The monkeys could walk on the other three legs; laboratory footage shows each dragging its useless limb behind.[41] The damage to the spinal cord meant that messages could not reach the limb—or became so dissipated that the signals were too weak to translate into movement. But that was before the monkeys had their brain waves *computerized*.

John Donoghue, in his earlier cursor experiments, had used elec-trodes to capture electrical brain signals, and then fed those signals into an algorithm, a finite sequence of well-defined, computer-implementable instructions. An external computer then decoded the mathematics into commands that the patients could also understand, though un-fortunately never quite as simply as "move the arm." It required training the patient as well as the machine. In this new experiment, however,

Borton intended to go much further that any human studies had done. In some ways, it was also simpler. Matthew Nagle had to train himself to understand the codes and commands given by the computer, then learn how to get his own brain to send signals back that would make sense to that interface; there was no one-to-one translation of a simple thought like "I'll grab it" into motion, just weeks of trial and error. Here the connection would be more direct. Electrodes would be implanted as before to capture the brain's signal: *Move the leg.* Also as before, an external computer would decode these signals into commands, but this time the monkey need not try to understand them, nor learn to think them back into the loop. Instead, the computer sent the signal directly to additional electrodes in the lumbar spine, completing the circuit from motor cortex to limb. They *bypassed* the site of the injury, but they also bypassed the conscious need to translate commands (i.e., moving a joystick cursor or an artificial limb).[42] In essence, the brain and the leg now worked as they had before—by skipping the problems of the neural superhighway and taking a detour.

The monkeys in Borton's study took to the technology "effortlessly." They didn't even turn around to examine the once-estranged leg—"they just walked."[43] Borton and his team had taken the monkeys' natural movement commands from brain to leg, and they had done it without bothering to fix the spinal cord: they just hopped over the gap. Borton and his team called this the brain-spine interface. Another scientist on the study, Grégoire Courtine, warned that this sort of tech wouldn't be available for humans just yet; for one thing, bipedal animals operate very differently from four-legged ones. But the day *was* coming. His work continued at the Swiss Federal Institute of Technology in Lausanne, and he had just invited three *human* participants to take part in a trial: Sebastian Tobler, Gertjan Oskan, and David Mzee.

Everything began with surgery. Courtine took Borton's protocol as inspiration, implanting a small patch of electrodes on the surface of the spinal cord in the lower back, below the injury. He then wired the electrodes to an internal pacemaker device that could be triggered to deliver bursts of electrical stimulation to individual muscles as they were called into use.[44] Unlike the monkey surgery, however, Courtine avoided implants in the human brain. He aimed instead for *targeted* stimulation, turning the device on and then using pulses of stimulus to coincide with intended movement. In other words, if you wanted to lift your left leg, you sent a pulse at the moment your brain signaled that it should move. All three participants had been chosen because their injuries still allowed some electrical signals to pass from brain to body. The brain's signal was too weak to reach the leg, but the shock would arrive at roughly the same time. What Courtine proposed wasn't a leap over the connection gap, but a signal booster; the device, when turned on, amplified electrical signals from the brain to the desired limbs. It took months of physical therapy and training before the patients could make their first awkward steps—jerking, ungainly motion with the support of crutches and stabilizers. But they were *walking*.

Then, months after he'd begun using the device, Mzee awoke in the middle of the night to a tickling sensation on his left side. It was his toe. He'd been moving it in his sleep—without the device. He thought at first he'd dreamed it, but with concentration, he found he could move it again, wiggling it back and forth on his brain's own commands.[45] Bit by bit, more control returned; he extended his knee and flexed his hip. In five months, he could take a few steps on his own, without the device.

This was completely unexpected.[46] "What we observed in animals is that it seems that the nerve fibers are regrowing and reconnecting the brain to the spinal cord," Courtine explained. Of course, some of this had been seen before in mice—yet in mice and rats and other small mammals, some regrowth appears even in control groups who hadn't been stimulated at all. It was thought that their simpler neural networks, coupled with their quadrupedal gait, accounted for this sort of progress, but no one had anticipated it happening in the more complex human animal. Though Mzee saw the greatest improvement, Oskan would regain some motor control, too—and Tobler could eventually get back on a modified bike powered by the combined motion of his arms and legs.[47] Newspapers and journals hailed it as a near miracle, as though Nuveen's Christopher Reeve commercial had finally come to life. In 2019, Mzee walked across the start line of the Wings for Life charity run, raising funds for spinal research. He would keep it up for thirty minutes, covering a quarter mile, to the astonished cheers of thousands.

But there was a catch. As with all scientific endeavors, a word of caution remains: *Don't believe the hype.* The targeting device could not offer continuous stimulation or muscles became confused; after all, the patient needed to think about picking up and putting down their feet. Timing was critical and needed to coincide with the desire to walk and move—and no device can outpace the lightning-fast response of the brain. Uncomfortable for long-term use, and far too expensive and unreliable for use outside a lab setting, Courtine's miracle device ultimately demonstrated *possibility* rather than enacting a cure. None of the men could walk very far without the device turned on; even Mzee didn't perform his quarter mile without aid. Back in Ohio at Case Western Research University, Dr. Kim Anderson, professor of physical medicine and rehabilitation, remained cautious. "We're still a long way from people being able to access this as standard medical care," she warned.[48] The benefit of BrainGate's unique multi-university, multinational approach, however, was its breadth. Courtine's design wasn't the only one available. At the University of California, Irvine, biomedical engineer Zoran Nenadic and neurologist An Do decided to attempt

Borton's original monkey study in a human being: not just stimulating muscles, but allowing the brain to leap over the gap.

Cybernetic technology has been a trope of science fiction for far longer than it's been a reality. Darth Vader, for instance, couldn't survive without his own externalized system to regulate his signature breathing, and in the science fiction film *Elysium*, Matt Damon's protagonist opts to have a surgically implanted exoskeleton to enable his radiation-weakened body to move with speed and agility. When *Elysium* released in 2013, the website Live Science compared the film's medical/military tech to BrainGate, embedding links in the article to tales of Courtine's early experiments in electronic stimulation. The new Irvine study, however, would dispense with Borton's and Courtine's surgical methods in favor of EEG.

The trial's sole subject, a man who had been paralyzed for five years, wore an EEG-activated "cap" to measure brain activity without embedded electrodes.[49] He then *thought about walking*. His first efforts were akin to moonwalks, done while suspended in the air. But after extensive physical therapy, the patient donned his electrode cap at the start of a 12-foot course and went through the motions of using his legs. The brain fired commands, which sped through a computer in nanoseconds and triggered external electrodes placed at the knee and wired to his EEG cap. Like Borton's monkey, but without a single surgical stitch, a paralyzed human being walked for the first time without using his spinal cord at all. It required a suspension harness, parallel bars for arm support, and many thousands of dollars in equipment—but it was a start.

The question remains: What if we don't need the spinal cord? What if we could, like characters of science fiction, bypass the injuries we sustained to our spines? Might that mean the recipients of White's cephalic transplant, which completely severed all spinal tissue, could ultimately overcome their paralysis? And would that be enough to make the surgery—in the end, not much more expensive than many of the BrainGate studies—viable, even desirable? "Yes, much of this theory is still science fiction," White would write in one of his last *News-Herald* columns. But so much science fiction had already come to pass, from face transplants to mechanical hearts that plug into wall outlets to recharge. About forty patients worldwide had received "new" hands; White had even met one of them, a German policeman who'd lost both his own while trying to defuse a bomb.[50] White had been in southern Germany for a holiday, and the man had arrived for their appointment on a motorcycle, a machine that required far more dexterity to operate than the steering wheel of a car. He proudly shook White's hand, with a hand that had not originally been his own.[51]

"[PBS] *NOVA* has contacted me," White continued in his article, because they wanted his opinion on whether damaged parts of a brain could be replaced the way hands were. It's true some experiments had been attempted, including the transplant of (non-brain) fetal tissue into the brains of Parkinson's patients. Alas, White assured PBS, the answer was no. "In spite of thousands of scientific reports, not one [of the brain section replacement] experiments has ever been successfully done," White explained—*but* a full-body transplant *had* been done. By White, of course, on monkeys. "The importance of [my] achievement has already been hailed throughout the world," he wrote, even if it had never been performed on human beings.[52] There were some bridges no one was yet ready to cross. White ended the column with the same claim he'd made since the beginning, the reason he'd become a neurologist in the first place: "Remember, brain tissue is the most complex and sophisticated matter in this world"—always and ever, for White, the repository of all we are.[53]

The article appeared on August 22, 2010. It would be White's last. Still awaiting news from the Nobel Prize committee, the surgeon-scientist began to fail. His body had never fully recovered from his accident, and he'd begun to suffer the effects of diabetes and a slow-moving prostate cancer. His mind, once so alert, began to cloud over. He dictated last letters to his daughter, and through her, attempted to put the final touches on what he hoped might be his memoirs. But a month after his final written piece ran in the pages of the *News-Herald*, Robert J. White died at home, on the shores of the lake, a stone's throw from the beach where his children and grandchildren played. The day was September 16, 2010; he was eighty-four.

The Nobel Prize in medicine would be awarded in October, but by a long-standing rule, it could not be earned posthumously. The prize went to Robert G. Edwards for his work on in vitro fertilization.

No one, not even Dr. White, can live forever. But Murray was right: White's contributions to deep hypothermia are still having profound clinical effects in modern trauma wards and neurosurgery. Today, therapeutic hypothermia saves cardiac arrest patients from cellular death in the brain, and extensive deep-brain surgery makes use of the ability to put the brain in a kind of stasis where it doesn't demand oxygen and stays safe from damage.[54] White's split-hemisphere surgeries now inform studies of the brain's response to everything from insulin to estrogen.[55] White laid the foundation for studies in neuroplasticity and even the ethics of brain death.[56] But he remains best known for doing the one thing considered unthinkable by even the most daring of his peers. Only a butcher would be so base as to repeat the trials of Frankenstein; only a man invested in the preservation of life and a belief in the transcendent soul would do it for reasons so strangely benevolent. To the last, he remained convinced that the surgery *would* be performed, somewhere, someday, and that his work would be exonerated.

# CONCLUSION

## Dr. Frankenstein's Reprise

*I*n Frankenstein, *the creature speaks to Victor of the horror of his being; he calls* himself an abortion, a thing that ought not to exist. The novel does not imagine a *before*. Mary Shelley considered her monster a blank slate, an empty vessel that must learn everything anew, even identity. And yet Victor Frankenstein used an adult brain, a processing unit that must have been complete in some other body, somewhere else, and the film adaptations make much of that possibility. What would it mean to awake as yourself but in a new body, to look through your own eyes and see something strange and unfamiliar? It speaks to us of horror, for estranged embodiment disturbs us far more than monstrosity. It reminds us just how much we rely on this body of ours—such a part of the identity we practice from the earliest stages of childhood. And yet when the body turns against us, would the transplant of the brain be so different from any other means of preserving our fragile human lives?

White once said that coming up with the head transplant might have been the worst thing he did for his career, that perhaps too near a connection to Shelley's *Frankenstein* had kept him from the accolades a half century of successful surgery ought to have delivered.[1] But scientific exploration can be, at times, like a river running underground. An idea disappears for a while, only to turn up again in the most unlikely of places, and sometimes with surprising force. Three years after Dr. White's death, an unusual paper appeared in *Surgical Neurology International*, a peer-reviewed medical journal based in the United States. The piece was written by a surgeon named Sergio Canavero, of the Turin Advanced Neuromodulation Group in Italy, and it boasted an unusual title: "HEAVEN: The Head Anastomosis Venture."

The article begins with Robert White's 1970 monkey cephalic transplant. Canavero blames the lack of support for head transplants on science's inability to heal the spinal cord.[2] If only the cord could be regenerated, if only the superhighway of information could be reconnected, then surely, Canavero reasons, head transplants would rise again. This assessment might miss the ethical conundrums that also plagued White, or the difficulty he faced in receiving permission and funding, but Canavero would soon become famous for brushing aside such doubts. Science was about *can*, he asserted, not *should*. "Should" was society's problem, not his—he was "just the technician," and as such, his role was to engineer solutions.[3]

"What follows," Canavero wrote in that 2013 article, proposing how a human head transplant might work, "is a possible scenario in order to give the reader a feel for the whole endeavor."[4] The description repeats White's surgical protocol from *Scientific American*, even quoting directly in several places: "The two teams, working in concert, would make deep incisions around each patient's neck, carefully separating all the anatomical structures to expose the carotid and vertebral arteries, jugular veins and spine" being one example. Canavero even provides White's concluding words from the article, where he speaks of a future where head transplants will be commonplace. For Canavero, White's words were predictive, and Canavero himself would be the first to make them a reality through a new technology for "fixing" a broken spine. He called this extraordinary procedure GEMINI, or *cord anastomosis*.[5] The secret to its success (he claimed) would be fusogens, the "brain glue" of Harold Hillman's dreams.

## GLUE, GOO, AND POLYETHYLENE GLYCOL

Harold Hillman was always fond of glue; he'd been speaking about it since the 1970s, often nudging along the idea that his work and White's would be complementary (White does not seem to have entirely agreed*). In October 2000, Hillman told Britain's *The Week* that he'd been working on a special "brain glue," a substance that would hold severed spinal cords together and allow them to regenerate. He proposed ingredients such as nerve growth factor, embryo extract, stem cells, tissue cultures, steroids, neuroglia, and vitamins. The work, however, remained mostly theoretical; he could not obtain funds to go on.[6] As a result of his controversial theories about brain cells (that there were only two types, not four, and that what other scientists thought they saw under electron microscopes was simply mistaken), he lost his credibility at the University of Surrey in the UK. They forced him into early retirement, even though he had served as director of the university's Unity Laboratory of Applied Neurobiology since 1970. It seemed glue had met a dead end. But like Frankenstein's monster, it would rise again—in 2003.

---

*In interviews, White only very tentatively referred to Hillman's glue idea. It wasn't entirely dismissal, but White didn't hold out the same hopes, as he'd not seen any proof that such a compound would really work.

Shai Shaham, head of a New York laboratory studying glial cells in roundworms, had made a surprising discovery. Making up 90 percent of brain structure, glial cells had long been thought of as mere support for more important parts of the brain: the neurons. But somehow, without appearing to have any organizational structure of their own, glial cells were responsible for organizing everything *else*. It appeared that glia (from the Greek word for "glue") had the ability to create boundaries and compartments, a means of shaping and separating the gelatinous gray matter we know as the brain. Exactly how far those generative properties might go remained a mystery—but opened doors for exploration. After damage to the spinal cord, glial cells formed into "scars" in the tissue; that much could be seen in the roundworms, but also in mice. What exactly did the scarring do? And what did it mean for spinal cord regeneration?

In 2004, a research team at the University of Melbourne isolated and blocked a molecule called EPHA4, thought to produce scar tissue around damaged spinal nerves by activating cells known as astrocytes.[7] The researchers selectively bred a group of mice without the molecule, then produced a spinal injury that paralyzed each mouse's left hind limb. Within three weeks, the mice redeveloped appropriate stride length, and in a month, the use of their ankles and toes.[8] Upon autopsy, the team discovered that spinal nerves had regrown across the damaged sections. It appeared, at first, to be an astounding breakthrough: *new spinal cords for everyone!* But the results had a few surprising complications. For one, even mice without the molecule recovered about 70 percent of their mobility. Geoffrey Raisman, director of the new spinal repair unit at University College London, dismissed the work because small animals frequently do get better all on their own—and the leap from mouse to man is hardly much closer than the jump from roundworms. Even so, work on regenerating spinal cords in mice and rats began in earnest, and soon a comprehensive study would be led at Case Western Reserve University, in the lab of Dr. Jerry Silver (who had previously argued against White's head transplant work). The different teams were relying, to varying degrees, on the abilities of the spinal cord itself and its glial glue. But at a lab in Purdue University, a new goo was on the horizon.

"Hope for Canine, Human Spinal Injuries" read the *Purdue University News* headline in the last days of 2004. Beneath it, a photo of a mustachioed professor of applied neuroscience and a caramel-colored dachshund named Kady. The project had begun five years earlier, on the eve of the new millennium; Richard Borgens and his partner, Riyi Shi, had been working on a literal guinea pig, trying to fuse nerve fibers together in its spinal cord. They did not use Hillman's recipe for "brain glue," instead opting for an actual liquid polymer known as polyethylene glycol (PEG).[9] Most people encounter PEG in its less-than-glamorous functions as a laxative or "personal lubricant," or in industrial applications as an ingredient in solvents, binders, and insulators. Borgens decided to inject PEG into the spinal cord at the site of injury, relying on the polymer's plasticlike qualities to fill gaps in ruptured cell membranes. His team discovered that cells could survive the initial traumatic rupture, but because damaged membranes failed to carry nerve impulses from one cell to the next, the cells tended to self-destruct. "Worse yet," Borgens wrote after the initial publication of his findings, chemicals seeping out of the dying cells sent "suicide signals" to the undamaged cells, causing a chain reaction of death and leading to irreparable spinal cord damage.[10] Borgens wasn't trying to *regrow* the cells; rather, he wanted the PEG glue to fix the membranes, allowing the cells to heal on their own.

The glue offered no cure for past spinal injuries, the membranes having been long ago destroyed. Borgens envisioned a day when every ambulance would keep a supply of PEG so that it might be administered immediately after injury to prevent paralysis in the first place. But this limited utility would not help a head transplant, with its wholly severed spinal cord—and Dr. White, who had known of the PEG studies, never considered it a real possibility. New techniques, however, were showing some surprising signs.

By the time Canavero's article appeared in 2013, graduate students in China had severed a rodent's spinal cord with diamond blades, then flooded the area with PEG. Two days later, the mouse could walk. The success was repeated on several continents—even in Dr. Silver's lab at Case Western Reserve University. But the director of Harbin Medical University hospital in northeastern China had plans for scaling up. Xiaoping Ren, though born in China, had worked with a team in Louisville, Kentucky, that performed the first hand transplant. After returning to China, he decided to try a more ambitious surgery—though on a smaller subject. He swapped the heads of a black mouse and a white mouse. Soon, he received correspondence from Canavero. Dr. Silver might contend that PEG success in mice didn't necessarily scale up; mice and humans certainly weren't equivalent beings. That did not deter Canavero in the least. His proposal to Ren was a simple one: Would he like to try the transplant on humans? Would his lab in Harbin be willing to host such a groundbreaking surgery? Canavero needed the lab and equipment Ren could supply—and China's comparatively lenient rules about surgical innovation. Canavero could provide his HEAVEN and GEMINI protocols, of course. But he also had something even more important. He had his first human volunteer.

The Atlantic carried the story under the headline "Audacious Plan to Save This Man's Life by Transplanting His Head." The featured photograph reveals a study in contrasts. Light filters through vertical blinds to fall upon the wistful features of a man in a crisp collared shirt. The profile is stark: a proud forehead and aquiline nose, chin held high. But where the light gives way to shadow, there is a wheelchair and only the merest hint of a body, wasted by disease. Valery Spiridonov, of Russia, suffered from Werdnig-Hoffmann disease, a genetic disorder that destroys muscle and kills the neurons that help the body move.[11] The condition is fatal in the end; the body literally wastes away to nothing. At thirty-one, Spiridonov ran an educational software company from his home. His entrepreneurial spirit might be compared to that of Craig Vetovitz, White's perfect patient, but the two had more than technological aspirations in common. Spiridonov had seen television footage of White during the surgeon's last visit to Ukraine, and heard of his plans for a head transplant. *That is the way,* he'd thought at the time. Spiridonov had never been able to run or walk, never gotten out of his wheelchair. A new body, a healthy body, seemed the best way to solve his troubles and extend his life. Spiridonov never had the chance to meet White, who had died a few years later. So when he saw Sergio Canavero in his (now infamous) TED Talk, he searched out his contact information and sent Canavero an email. If Canavero could do what he promised, then Spiridonov wanted to be the first volunteer.

Canavero's talk, which has garnered over half a million views, appeared in 2015. It also earned him epithets; critics called him "delusional," a "James Bond villain," and of course "Dr. Frankenstein."[12] The fifty-two-year-old Italian surgeon stepped onto the stage with a shaved head, in a turtleneck and jeans, like a surgical Steve Jobs. "All the experts know is wrong," he announced. "Sit tight, I'm about to give you one hell of a ride."[13] The talk, later flagged by the TED organization for not following their "curatorial guidelines"* (and probably because they believed his findings impossible), ranges from promises of spinal fusing to the thinly veiled suggestion that billionaires in Russia could live forever if they cloned enough bodies to swap heads with. Canavero swaggers with unmistakable bravado, proudly asserting his authorship of a book on "female seduction"; viewers learn he doesn't eat beef, practices jujitsu, and likes to talk about his six-pack.[14] But he also successfully introduced cortical brain stimulation for Parkinson's (a process by which motor nerves are magnetically stimulated deep in the brain), has written textbooks on dysfunction of the central nervous system, and has author or coauthor credits for over one hundred peer-reviewed publications. And it is clear that he believes his version of the White Surgery will work.

Canavero intends to build his operating theater complete with a crane, so that the head can be "floated" to the donor body, where their stumps would be aligned, PEG employed, and electrical stimulus given to (supposedly) help establish communication across the severed spinal cord.[15] Reattachment would be more labored than in White's monkey surgeries, as all muscle tissues and nerves would have to be reknit together. White hadn't bothered; it didn't matter much without the spinal cord to direct nerve impulses. And even Canavero doesn't expect the nerves and muscles to work again straightaway. The body must be tethered to life support until signs of motor recovery appear. Spiridonov might move his eyes or lips, the same tickling returns of life

---

*The note from TED reads: "We've flagged this talk, which was filmed at an independent TEDx event, because it appears to fall outside TEDx's curatorial guidelines. This talk is best viewed as a speculative what-if scenario, and with awareness that the 2017 surgeries performed by Dr. Canavero on human cadavers have raised practical and ethical concerns in the scientific community. The talk contains statements about nerve regeneration that are questioned by many neuroscientists."

White watched for in his monkey surgery all those years before.[16] But the surgeons would also be watching for the curl of a toe, the clutch of a hand. The surgery, Canavero claimed, has a "90 percent plus" chance of success—though his colleague Ren made no such promises.[17]

In 2016, Canavero replicated White's monkey surgery and published photos of the primate, its neck zipper-stitched together where it lay against a white towel. "We'll do it on humans next year," he promised, around Christmas. "It's no longer 'loony Sergio,'" he exclaimed in an interview with Canada's *National Post*. "Now, we are many loonies around the world working on this."[18] It may have been something of an overstatement; most neurosurgeons were no more impressed by Canavero's claims than White's own.

Christmas 2017 came and went. So with 2018 and 2019. Permission from the Chinese government was not quite as easily managed as Canavero first implied, though no reasons for the stall were given. He also lost his test case. Spiridonov met and married his wife, Anastasia, in 2018, and with the birth of their son, he canceled his part in the HEAVEN transplant project. Spiridonov's wife had no interest in the surgery anyway. People like Spiridonov, she said, "are much deeper, feeling, faithful, kind-hearted, and also they are usually very smart. Isn't that the main thing?"[19] Spiridonov followed up with *Good Morning Britain* from his new home in Florida. "In my life appeared a woman who I fell in love with," he told the newscasters happily.[20] With so many reasons to live just as he is, Spiridonov decided he wasn't interested in experiments that might be merely "expensive euthanasia."[21]

Dr. White had insisted all along that every life was worth living. Paralysis wasn't the end. Even his work with Craig Vetovitz had been motivated by the latter's potential loss of kidney function, though in an ironic twist, Craig lived seven years longer than White himself. Yet the hope for a head transplant nevertheless contains a concurrent hope for permanence, even immortality. If parts could be replaced endlessly, if brains could be sustained infinitely, what would that mean? Canavero's throwaway comment about Russian billionaires is telling. Body transplants, if ever they arrive, are the province of privilege. An article in the journal *Futurism* complained that "only men would be stupid enough to believe that bodies were transferrable. It is part of their privilege . . . As though that body is an accessory, rather than an integral aspect of personhood . . . As though their quirks and chemical detritus isn't written on every crease of our mind."[22] Our bodies are not singular entities, but whole universes of microbes and bacteria working in concert with cellular activity; we may not be what we eat, exactly, but the gut alone has been proven to influence the brain in surprising ways—from mood to pain response. What would a head transplant really accomplish? Would it rearrange, enhance, or obliterate the "self"? Would it rewrite the rules of death? Or would it become, like so many other technologies, just another way for the "haves" to have more?

White had been a Cartesian at heart, believing in the division between mind and body, soul and matter, even if the truth that most of us encounter is far messier. For White, the transplant surgery was a puzzle, an impossibility that could be overturned by the scientific mind. But it may have been something more, too. It may have been the best way to align his two guiding principles, his two primary motivators: science . . . and God. Were White able to achieve the head transplant, it would certainly have given him a place among the greatest breakthrough scientists of our time. It might have sealed his reputation in ways even his bid for the Nobel Prize failed to do. White, the surgeon, could hold the living brain in his hands . . . the proof of life after bodily death. The soul, the self, the intangible holy grail of so many philosophers, theologians, and medical giants: Was that not something for White to aim for?

White had concluded his 1999 article on the bionic future with the following quote: "I predict that what has always been the stuff of science fiction—the Frankenstein legend, in which an entire human being is constructed by sewing various body parts together—will become a clinical reality early in the 21st century."[23] Twenty years on, in March 2019, Ren and Canavero published two articles claiming they'd fully transected the spinal cords of monkeys and dogs, then put them back together again. Both studies, published in *Surgical Neurology International*, claimed the animals could walk after the surgery, supported by video evidence.[24] The story broke in *USA Today*, and a follow-up exchange with Ren suggested that the findings were proof that human trials should be initiated. Despite all the setbacks, White's words for the new millennium might still prove prophetic.

The quest to transplant the soul continues on.

FINIS

# *Notes*

## CHAPTER 1: FOR WANT OF A KIDNEY

1. Nicholas L. Tilney, *Transplant: From Myth to Reality* (New Haven, CT: Yale University Press, 2003), 37.
2. Ann Rooney, *The History of Medicine* (New York: Rosen Publishing, 2012), 154.
3. Tilney, *Transplant*, 37.
4. David Hamilton, *The First Transplant Surgeon: The Flawed Genius of Nobel Prize Winner Alexis Carrel* (Hackensack, NJ: World Scientific, 2016), 110–11.
5. Susan E. Lederer, *Flesh and Blood: Organ Transplantation and Blood Transfusion in Twentieth-Century America* (New York: Oxford University Press, 2008), 7.
6. Ibid., 7.
7. Tilney, *Transplant*, 17.
8. Ibid., 7.
9. New York biologist Leo Loeb, quoted in Tilney, 37.
10. Tilney, 98.
11. Ibid.
12. National Institute of Diabetes and Digestive and Kidney Disease, https://www.niddk.nih.gov/.
13. Joseph E. Murray, *Surgery of the Soul: Reflections on a Curious Career* (Sagamore Beach, MA: Science History Publications, 2001), 73.
14. Ibid., 75.
15. Joseph E. Murray, "The Fight for Life: The Pioneering Surgeon of the World's First Successful Human Organ Transplant Reflects on the Gift of Life," *Harvard*

*Medicine*, Autumn 2019, https://hms.harvard.edu/magazine/science-emotion/fight -life.

16. Joseph E. Murray, interview by Martin Woolf, *On the Beat*, New York Organ Donor Network publication, May 25, 2004.

17. Pacific Immunology, "Antibody Introduction: What Is an Antibody?," accessed September 5, 2019, https://www.pacificimmunology.com/resources/antibody -introduction/what-is-an-antibody/.

18. Murray, *Surgery of the Soul*, 16.

19. "Francis Daniels Moore Dies at 88," *Harvard Gazette*, December 6, 2001.

20. Joseph E. Murray, "Remembrances of the Early Days of Renal Transplantation," *Transplantation Proceedings* 13, suppl. 1 (February 1981): 9–15.

21. James Renner, "White's Anatomy," *Cleveland Free Times*, March 7, 2007.

22. Andy Hollandbeck, Jeff Nilsson, and Demaree Bess, "Not So Neutral: America's War Efforts before Pearl Harbor," *Saturday Evening Post*, August 11, 2016.

23. "Army Battle Casualties and Nonbattle Deaths in World War II," Combined Arms Research Library, Department of the Army, June 25, 1953, https://apps.dtic.mil /dtic/tr/fulltext/u2/a438106.pdf.

24. Laura Putre, "The Frankenstein Factor: Cleveland Brain Surgeon Robert J. White Has a Head for Transplanting," *Cleveland Scene*, December 9, 1999, https://www .clevescene.com/cleveland/the-frankenstein-factor/Content?oid=1473264.

25. Murray, *Surgery of the Soul*, 80–81.

26. Ibid., 80.

27. Ibid.

28. Ibid., 81.

29. Ibid.

30. Ibid.

31. Ibid., 119.

32. Ibid., 120.

33. Putre, "The Frankenstein Factor."

## CHAPTER 2: TWO-HEADED DOGS AND THE SPACE RACE

1. Simon Matskeplishvili, "Vladimir Petrovich Demikhov (1916–1998): A Pioneer of Transplantation Ahead of His Time, Who Lived Out the End of His Life as an Unknown and in Poor Circumstances," *European Heart Journal* 38, no. 46 (December 7, 2017): 3406–10, https://doi.org/10.1093/eurheartj/ehx697.

2. "Envoys Stalk Again as Nikita Rants," *Milwaukee Sentinel*, November 19, 1956.

3. Quoted from Khrushchev's "We Will Bury You," February 7, 1962, Central Intelligence Agency, approved for release January 4, 2002, accessed March 25, 2019,

https://www.cia.gov/library/readingroom/document/cia-rdp73b00296r0002000
40087-1.

4. Audra J. Wolfe, *Competing with the Soviets: Science, Technology, and the State in Cold War America* (Baltimore: Johns Hopkins Press, 2013), 9.

5. Ibid., 9.

6. Ibid., 19.

7. Ibid., 18.

8. Ibid.

9. Wolfe, *Competing with the Soviets*, 20.

10. Mark Popovsky, *Science in Chains: The Crisis of Science and Scientists in the Soviet Union*, trans. Paula S. Falla (London: Collins and Harvill Press, 1980), 23.

11. Wolfe, *Competing with the Soviets*, 55.

12. Robert White, interview by Paul Copeland, director, in *Stranger than Fiction: The First Head Transplant* (UK: ITN Factual, 2006).

13. Ibid.

14. Larry Greenemeier, "US and Soviet Spooks Studied Paranormal Powers to Find a Cold War Advantage," *NewsBlog, Scientific American*, October 20, 2008.

15. I. E. Konstantinov, "A Mystery of Vladimir P. Demikhov: The 50th Anniversary of the First Intrathoracic Transplantation," *Annals of Thoracic Surgery* 65 (1998): 1171–77, DOI: 10.1016/S0003-4975(97)01308-8.

16. I. E. Konstantinov, "At the Cutting Edge of the Impossible: A Tribute to Vladimir P. Demikhov," *Texas Heart Institute Journal* 36, no. 5 (2009): 453–58.

17. Matskeplishvili, "Vladimir Petrovich Demikho," 3406.

18. Konstantinov, "A Mystery of Vladimir P. Demikhov."

19. Matskeplishvili, "Vladimir Petrovich Demikhov," 3406.

20. Ibid., 3407.

21. Konstantinov, "At the Cutting Edge of the Impossible."

22. Konstantinov, "A Mystery of Vladimir P. Demikhov."

23. Ibid.

24. R. M. Langer, "Vladimir P. Demikhov, a Pioneer of Organ Transplantation," *Transplant Proceedings* 43 (2011): 1221–22.

25. Wolfe, *Competing with the Soviets*, 40.

26. Michael D'Antonio, *A Ball, a Dog, and a Monkey: 1957—The Space Race Begins* (New York: Simon & Schuster, 2007), 5.

27. Quoted in D'Antonio, 14.

28. Quoted in D'Antonio, 15.

29. D'Antonio, 42.

30. Ibid., 25.

31. Quoted in D'Antonio, 36.

32. Associated Press, "Edmund Stevens, 81, a Reporter in Moscow for 40 Years, Is Dead," *New York Times*, May 27, 1992.

33. Ibid.

34. Edmund Stevens, "How Shavka Joined Brodyaga," *Life* 47, no. 3 ( July 20, 1959).

35. Ibid.

36. Ibid.

37. From the description and photo evidence provided in Stevens, "How Shavka Joined Brodyaga."

38. Vladimir Demikhov, quoted in Stevens, "How Shavka Joined Brodyaga."

39. "History of the Kidney Disease Treatment," St. George's Kidney Patients Association, https://www.sgkpa.org.uk/main/history-of-the-kidney-disease-treatment.

40. Quoted in Stevens, "How Shavka Joined Brodyaga."

41. Ibid.

42. Mark, "I've Been Working in the Kremlin with a Two-Headed Dog," *Galileo's Doughnuts* (blog), *Medium*, May 6, 2015, https://medium.com/galileos-doughnuts/i-ve-been-working-in-the-kremlin-with-a-two-headed-dog-eb29132466dc.

43. "Russia's Two-Headed Dog," *Life* 47, no. 3 ( July 20, 1959).

44. Robert White, interview, in James Renner, "White's Anatomy," *Cleveland Free Times*, March 7, 2007.

45. Ibid.

46. Walt Tomford, phone interview with the author, July 19, 2018.

47. White, in Renner, "White's Anatomy."

48. Howard Yonas, phone interview with the author, August 13, 2018; George Dakters, phone interview with the author, July 17, 2018.

49. White, in *Stranger than Fiction*.

50. Sam Kean, *The Tale of the Dueling Neurosurgeons* (New York: Back Bay Books, 2014), 256.

51. Sunil Manjila et al., "From Hypothermia to Cephalosomatic Anastomoses: The Legacy of Robert White (1926–2010) at Case Western Reserve University of Cleveland," *World Neurosurgery* 113 (May 2018): 14–25.

52. Stacey Conradt, "The Quick Eight," Mental Floss, February 11, 2009.

53. Henry Gully, "History of Accidental Hypothermia," *Resuscitation* 82, no. 1 (2011): 122–25.

54. Robert Falcon Scott, quoted in Gully.

55. John Bryk et al., "Deep Brain Hypothermia by Means of High-Flow Biventricular Cooling," *Resuscitation* 5, no. 4 (1976–1977): 223–28.

56. Zawn Villines, "What Happens After a Lack of Oxygen to the Brain?" SpinalCord
    .com, June 13, 2016.
57. White, in Renner, "White's Anatomy."
58. Manjila et al., "From Hypothermia to Cephalosomatic Anastomoses."
59. Steven Johnson, *Where Good Ideas Come From: The Natural History of Innovation*,
    (New York: Riverhead Books, 2011), 45.
60. Wagner, "The Brain Research Laboratory at the Cleveland Metropolitan General
    Hospital and Case Western Reserve University," *Journal of Neurosurgery* 101, no. 4
    (2004): 881–87.
61. Walt Tomford, phone interview with the author, July 19, 2018.
62. Franklin C. Wagner Jr., "The Brain Research Laboratory," 881.
63. Ibid.
64. David Bennun, "Dr. Robert White," *Sunday Telegraph Magazine*, 2000, archived at
    https://www.bennun.biz/interviews/drwhite.html.
65. Wolfe, *Competing with the Soviets*, 91.
66. Ibid., 93.
67. Ibid., 94.
68. Ibid.
69. Ibid., 95.

## CHAPTER 3: WHAT DO DEAD BRAINS THINK?

1. Frank Hellinger, Byron Bloor, and John McCutchen, "Total Cerebral Blood Flow
   and Oxygen Consumption Using the Dye-Dilution Method: A Study of Occlu-
   sive Arterial Disease and Cerebral Infarction," *Journal of Neurosurgery* 19, no. 11
   (1962): 964.
2. Min Lang et al., "A Tribute to Dr. Robert J. White," *Neurosurgery* 85, no. 2 (2019):
   E366–73, DOI: 10.1093/neuros/nyy321.
3. Wagner, "The Brain Research Laboratory at the Cleveland Metropolitan General
   Hospital and Case Western Reserve University,": 881–87.
4. Ibid.
5. J. Verdura, R. J. White, and H. E. Kretchmer, "A Simplified Method for Obtaining
   Cerebrospinal Fluid Pressure Measurements in the Dog," *Journal of Applied Physiology* 18, no. 4 (1963): 837–38.
6. Wagner, "The Brain Research Laboratory."
7. Robert White, Maurice S. Albin, and Javier Verdura, "Isolation of the Monkey
   Brain: In vitro Preparation and Maintenance," *Science* 141, no. 3585 (September 13,
   1963): 1060–61.

8. Ibid.

9. Oriana Fallaci, "The Dead Body and the Living Brain," *Look*, November 28, 1967, 108.

10. David Donald and Robert White, "Selective Perfusion in the Monkey: Effects of Maintained Cerebral Hypothermia," *Journal of Surgical Research* 2, no. 3 (May 1962): 213–20.

11. Ibid., 218.

12. Sam Kean, *The Tale of the Dueling Neurosurgeons* (New York: Back Bay Books, 2014), 33.

13. Ibid., 8–9.

14. Michael White, interview with the author, Willoughby, Ohio, January 8, 2019.

15. Robert White, interview, in James Renner, "White's Anatomy," *Cleveland Free Times*, March 7, 2007.

16. Ibid.

17. White, Albin, and Verdura, "Isolation of the Monkey Brain," 1060.

18. Robert White, Maurice Albin, Javier Verdura, and George Locke, "The Isolated Monkey Brain: Operative Preparation and Design of Support Systems," presented at the meeting of the Harvey Cushing Society in Los Angeles, CA, April 1, 1964. Supported by U. S. Public Health Service Grant NB-03859. 215–216.

19. Ibid., 216–17.

20. Ibid.

21. Ibid., 224.

22. White, Albin, and Verdura, "Isolation of the Monkey Brain," 1061.

23. Leo Massopust, quoted in Alvin Toffler, *Future Shock* (New York: Bantam, 1990), 214.

24. White, Albin, and Verdura, "Isolation of the Monkey Brain," 1061.

25. Francys Subiaul et al., "Cognitive Imitation in 2-Year-Old Children (Homo sapiens): A Comparison with Rhesus Monkeys (*Macaca mulatta*)," *Animal Cognition* 10, no. 4 (2007): 369–75.

26. White et al., "The Isolated Monkey Brain," 216–17.

27. Ibid.

28. American Association of Neurological Surgeons, "History," https://www.aans.org/About-Us/History.

29. Harold M. Schmeck Jr., "Brains Are Kept Alive for Tests After Removal from Monkeys," *New York Times*, June 8, 1964.

30. Michael DeGeorgia, interview with the author, University Hospital, Cleveland, Ohio, August 7, 2018.

31. Eelco F. M. Wijdicks, *Brain Death*, 3rd ed. (Oxford: Oxford University Press, 2017).

32. Schmeck, "Brains Are Kept Alive."

33. Ibid.

34. Robert White, "Historical Development of Spinal Cord Cooling," *Surgical Neurology* 25, no. 3 (1986): 295–98.

35. Schmeck, "Brains Are Kept Alive."

36. Robert White, interview by Paul Copeland, director, in *Stranger than Fiction: The First Head Transplant.*

37. Michael White, interview with the author, Willoughby, Ohio, January 8, 2009.

38. White, in Renner, "White's Anatomy."

39. Patty White, interview, August 8, 2018.

40. Robert White, "Discovering the Pathway for Cooling the Brain," *Paths of Discovery,* acta 18 (Vatican City: Pontifical Academy of Sciences, 2006).

41. Harold Hillman, "Dr. Robert J. White (1926–2010)," *Resuscitation Journal* 83 (2012): 18–19.

## CHAPTER 4: BRAINS BEHIND THE IRON CURTAIN (OR, SCIENCE, VODKA, AND PRETTY GIRLS)

1. Peter Grose, "Soviet Overrules Its Scientists, Bars U. S. Research Ship's Visit," *New York Times,* May 21, 1966, 1, 27.

2. Ibid.

3. Harold Hillman, quoted in "Harold Hillman, Biological Scientist," obituary, *Telegraph,* September 7, 2016.

4. Robert White, interview by Paul Copeland, director, in *Stranger than Fiction: The First Head Transplant.*

5. United Press International, "2 Americans Held in Soviet Meet with Russian Lawyers," *New York Times,* November 27, 1966, accessed January 15, 2019, https://nyti.ms/2RNTShn.

6. United Press International, "Russian Republic Stiffens Laws Against 'Slanders,'" *New York Times,* October 6, 1966, accessed January 15, 2019, https://nyti.ms/2RNUe7H.

7. United Press International, "A Russian, in 494 Pages, Finds U.S. Life All Bad," *New York Times,* December 11, 1966, accessed January 15, 2019, https://nyti.ms/3aFIz1v.

8. Robert White, quoted in Laura Putre, "The Frankenstein Factor: Cleveland Brain Surgeon Robert J. White Has a Head for Transplanting," *Cleveland Scene,* December 9, 1999, https://www.clevescene.com/cleveland/the-frankenstein-factor/Content?oid=1473264.

9. Michael White, interview with the author, Willoughby, Ohio, January 7, 2019.

10. "Andrei P. Romodanov, MD, interviewed by Robert White, MD." Supported by the

American Association of Neurosurgeons, 9th European Conference of Neurosurgery, Moscow, 1991, https://www.youtube.com/watch?v=dPHi3VLo6JE.

11. Ibid.

12. Boleslav Lichterman, "A History of Russian and Soviet Neuro(path)ology," in *History of Neurology*, Stanley Finger, François Boller, and Kenneth L. Tyler, eds., vol. 95, 3rd series (Amsterdam: Elsevier, 2009), 746.

13. Joy Neumeyer, "A Visit to Moscow's Institute of the Brain," *Vice*, April 10, 2014, accessed January 17, 2019, https://www.vice.com/en_us/article/qbejbd/a-visit-to-moscows-brain-institute.

14. White, in *Stranger than Fiction*.

15. Harold Hillman, in *Stranger than Fiction*.

16. White, in *Stranger than Fiction*.

17. Gloria Stewart, "Life in Moscow in the Soviet 1960s: Memoirs of a British Journalist Part 1," *103rd Meridian East*, accessed January 17, 2019, http://meridian103.com/issue-14/history/moscow-in-the-soviets/.

18. Ibid.

19. Gloria Stewart, "Life in Moscow in the Soviet 1960s: Memoirs of a British Journalist Part 2," *103rd Meridian East*, accessed January 17, 2019, http://meridian103.com/issue-14/history/soviet-moscow/.

20. Michael White, interview with the author, January 7, 2019.

21. Mark Popovsky, *Science in Chains* (London: Collins Harvill, 1979), 3.

22. Quoted in Popovsky, 4.

23. Ibid., 5.

24. I. E. Konstantinov, "A Mystery of Vladimir P. Demikhov: The 50th Anniversary of the First Intrathoracic Transplantation," *Annals of Thoracic Surgery* 65 (1998): 1171–77, DOI: 10.1016 /S0003-4975(97)01308-8.

25. Quoted in Popovsky, 9.

26. Ibid., 11.

27. Ibid., 71.

28. Konstantinov, "A Mystery of Vladimir P. Demikhov: The 50th Anniversary of the First Intrathoracic Transplantation."

29. I. E. Konstantinov, "At the Cutting Edge of the Impossible: A Tribute to Vladimir P. Demikhov," *Texas Heart Institute Journal* 36, no. 5 (2009): 454.

30. Ibid.

31. Matskeplishvili, "Vladimir Petrovich Demikhov (1916–1998): A Pioneer of Transplantation Ahead of His Time, Who Lived Out the End of His Life as an Unknown and in Poor Circumstances."

32. Boleslav Lichterman, interview with author, the second Doctor as a Humanist conference, 2019.

33. Matskeplishvili, "Vladimir Petrovich Demikhov," 3407.

34. Konstantinov, "At the Cutting Edge of the Impossible."

35. Elena Berger et al., "The Unspoken History of Medicine in Russia," *MEDIC* 25, no. 2 (2017): 28–34.

36. Ibid., 31.

37. Konstantinov, "A Mystery of Vladimir P. Demikhov."

38. Eric Pace, "Vladimir P. Demikhov, 82, Pioneer in Transplants, Dies," *New York Times*, November 25, 1998, https://www.nytimes.com/1998/11/25/world/vladimir-p-demikhov-82-pioneer-in-transplants-dies.html.

39. White, in *Stranger than Fiction*.

40. Konstantinov, "A Mystery of Vladimir P. Demikhov."

41. Quoted in Carl Muller, "Swapping Heads and Brains—The Real-Life Frankenstein," *Saturday Magazine*, October 28, 2000, accessed January 24, 2019.

42. Robert White, interview, *Süddeutschen Zeitung*, August 25, 2000. Translated for *Southern Cross Review*, accessed January 24, 2019, https://www.southerncrossreview.org/8/transplant.html.

43. Robert White, interview, "Work Together for a Happier Life," *Moscow News*, June 1973, 23–30.

44. Ibid.

45. White, in *Stranger than Fiction*.

## CHAPTER 5: FRANKENSTEIN'S MONKEY

1. Oriana Fallaci, "The Dead Body and the Living Brain," *Look*, November 28, 1967, 100.

2. Ibid.

3. Ibid., 100–101.

4. Ibid., 101.

5. Ibid., 104.

6. Ibid., 105.

7. Ibid., 106.

8. Robert White, quoted in Fallaci, "The Dead Body and the Living Brain," 106.

9. Fallaci, "The Dead Body and the Living Brain," 106.

10. White, quoted in Fallaci, "The Dead Body and the Living Brain," 112.

11. Ibid.

12. Ibid.

13. Ibid.

14. Ibid.

15. Fallaci, "The Dead Body and the Living Brain," 104.

16. Ibid.

17. Lesley Sharp, *Animal Ethos: The Moralist of Human-Animal Encounters in Experimental Lab Science* (Oakland: University of California Press, 2019), 42–43.

18. Ibid., 42–44.

19. Ibid., 50.

20. Quoted in David Bennun, "Dr. Robert White," *Sunday Telegraph Magazine*, 2000, archived at https://www.bennun.biz/interviews/drwhite.html.

21. Ibid.

22. Christina DeStefano, "The Interview that Became Henry Kissinger's 'Most Disastrous Decision': How Oriana Fallaci Became the Most Feared Political Interviewer in the World," *Literary Hub*, October 2017; Judy Klemesrud, "Oriana Fallaci, an Interviewer Who Goes for the Jugular in Four Languages," *New York Times*, January 23, 1973.

23. Nina Burleigh, "Oriana Fallaci, Right or Wrong: Review of *Oriana Fallaci* by Christina DeStefano," *New York Times*, October 2017.

24. Fallaci, "The Dead Body and the Living Brain," 114.

25. Putre, "The Frankenstein Factor: Cleveland Brain Surgeon Robert J. White Has a Head for Transplanting."

26. Barbara Kleban, "A Devout Neurosurgeon Studies the Brain with Medically Dazzling, Morally Puzzling Head Transplants," *People*, August 13, 1979.

27. Ibid.

28. Robert White, quoted in Fallaci, "The Dead Body and the Living Brain," 106.

29. William Edward Addis and Thomas Arnold, *A Catholic Dictionary: Containing Some Account of the Doctrine, Discipline, Rites, Ceremonies, Councils, and Religious Orders of the Catholic Church* (London: Kegan Paul, Trench, Trübner, 1893), 851.

30. Quoted in Bennun, "Dr. Robert White."

31. Michael White and Patricia White, letter, February 2018.

32. Ibid.

33. Wagner, "The Brain Research Laboratory at the Cleveland Metropolitan General Hospital and Case Western Reserve University," 881–87.

34. Deborah Blum, *The Monkey Wars* (Oxford: Oxford University Press, 1994), 35–36.

35. Wagner, "The Brain Research Laboratory," 885.

36. Robert White et al., "Cephalic Exchange Transplantation in the Monkey," *Surgery* 70, no. 1 (1971): 135–39.

37. Ibid., 136.

38. Norman Taslitz, phone interview with the author, July 18, 2018.

39. White, "Discovering the Pathway for Cooling the Brain."

40. James Renner, "White's Anatomy," *Cleveland Free Times*, March 7, 2007.

41. Quoted in Bennun, "Dr. Robert White."

42. Patricia White, email, March 7, 2019.

43. White et al., "Cephalic Exchange Transplantation in the Monkey," 135–36.

44. Ibid., 136.

45. *Stranger than Fiction: The First Head Transplant*, Paul Copeland, director.

46. White et al., "Cephalic Exchange Transplantation in the Monkey," 135–36.

47. Quoted in Bennun, "Dr. Robert White."

48. *Stranger than Fiction*.

49. Robert White, interview in "A. Head B. Body," *Midnight Archive*, episode 05, special presentation, Jim Fields, director, 2008, 2011, YouTube, accessed March 7, 2019, https://www.youtube.com/watch?v=V2P-teoc2ic.

50. Quoted in Bennun, "Dr. Robert White."

51. Robert White, quoted in Putre, "The Frankenstein Factor."

52. White, interview in "A. Head B. Body."

53. White, quoted in Bennun, "Dr. Robert White."

54. Robert White, 1972 radio interview, quoted in "Head Transplant," *Motherboard*, July 9, 2013.

## CHAPTER 6: THE MODERN PROMETHEUS

1. Edgar Allan Poe, "The Premature Burial," quoted with thanks from Michael De-Georgia, "History of Brain Death as Death: 1968 to the Present," *Journal of Critical Care* 29, no. 4 (2014): 673–78.

2. Robert White, interview, "The Man Who Believes in Body Transplants," *Q.E.D.* (London: BBC Worldwide, 1989).

3. Margaret Locke, *Twice Dead: Organ Transplants and the Reinvention of Death* (Berkeley: University of California Press, 2001), 78.

4. Ibid.

5. Oriana Fallaci, "The Dead Body and the Living Brain," *Look*, November 28, 1967, 112.

6. DeGeorgia, "History of Brain Death as Death."

7. Locke, *Twice Dead*, 79.

8. Pope Pius XII, "The Prolongation of Life: An Address to an International Congress of Anaesthesiologists, November, 24 1957," *The Pope Speaks* 4, no. 4 (1958), 393–98.

9. DeGeorgia, "History of Brain Death as Death," 673.

10. Ibid., 675.

11. Raymond Hoffenberg, "Christiaan Barnard: His First Transplants and Their Impact on Concepts of Death," *BMJ* 323, no. 7327 (December 22, 2001): 1478–80.

12. DeGeorgia, "History of Brain Death as Death," 675.

13. Christiaan Barnard, "Surgical Innovation," *BMJ* 325, no. 7374 (November 23, 2002): 1195.

14. DeGeorgia, "History of Brain Death as Death," 675.

15. Ibid.

16. Robert White and Charles Curran, "The Morality of Human Transplants," *Sign* 47 (March 1968): 23.

17. Dennis Coday, "Charles Curran to Retire from Full-Time Teaching," *National Catholic Reporter*, May 15, 2014.

18. White and Curran, "The Morality of Human Transplants," 23.

19. Ibid.

20. Locke, *Twice Dead*, 78.

21. Hoffenberg, "Christiaan Barnard," 1478.

22. Ibid.

23. White and Curran, "The Morality of Human Transplants," 24.

24. Pope Pius XII, "The Prolongation of Life."

25. White and Curran, "The Morality of Human Transplants," 24.

26. Dr. Howard Yonas (previously White's resident), interview with the author, Cleveland Heights, Ohio, August 13, 2018.

27. White and Curran, "The Morality of Human Transplants," 23.

28. Ibid.

29. Ibid.

30. Hoffenberg, "Christiaan Barnard," 1479.

31. The nightmare scenario was described by an anonymous public health official in *Newsweek*, and also in H. A. Davidson, "Transplantation in the Brave New World," *Mental Hygiene* 52, no. 3 (July 1968): 467–68.

32. Maya Overby Koretzky, "'A Change of Heart': Racial Politics, Scientific Metaphor and Coverage of 1968 Interracial Heart Transplants in the African American Press," *Social History of Medicine* 30, no. 2 (May 2017): 408–28.

33. Robert M. Veatch, "Case Studies in Bioethics: Brain Death: Welcome Definition . . . or Dangerous Judgment?," *Hastings Center Report* 2, no. 5 (November 1972): 10–13.

34. Susan E. Lederer, "Putting Death in Context," *Hastings Center Report* 38, no. 6 (November–December 2008): 3, https://muse.jhu.edu/article/254294.

35. The case, to be decided in 1972, is recorded as: William E. Tucker, Administrator

of the Estate of Bruce O. Tucker, deceased, vs. Dr. Richard R. Lower, Dr. David M. Hume, Dr. David H. Sewell, Dr. H. M. Lee, and Dr. Abdullah Fatteh.

36. Harold Schmeck Jr., "Medicine," *New York Times*, June 4, 1972.

37. Barry Barkan, "Transplant Patient Is Impatient," *Baltimore Afro-American*, September 11, 1968; Koretzky, "'A Change of Heart.'"

38. Ibid.

39. Ibid.

40. Ibid.

41. Allen Howard, "With an Image of Nothing, He Created Man," *Cleveland Call & Post*, March 2, 1968. Quoted in Koretzky.

42. Kenneth L. Kusmer, "African Americans," *Encyclopedia of Cleveland History*, accessed May 1, 2019, https://case.edu/ech/articles/a/african-americans.

43. Emily Bamforth, "July 23 Marks 50-Year Anniversary of Glenville Riots," Cleveland.com, July 23, 2018.

44. Ibid.

45. Ibid.

46. Locke, *Twice Dead*, 91.

47. Quoted in Koretzky, "'A Change of Heart.'"

48. Christiaan Barnard, quoted in Locke, *Twice Dead*.

49. Locke, *Twice Dead*, 97.

50. Dennis Kucinich (OH), Selections from "Honoring the Life and Achievements of His Holiness Pope John Paul II and Expressing Profound Sorrow on His Death," *Congressional Record* 151, no. 38 (April 6, 2005): H1807–21.

51. Ibid.

52. James Renner, "White's Anatomy," *Cleveland Scene*, March 7, 2007.

53. Robert White, quoted in Renner, "White's Anatomy."

54. Marcelo Sanchez Sorondo, "Introduction," in *Papal Addresses to the Pontifical Academy of Sciences 1917–2002* (Vatican City: Pontifical Academy of Sciences, 2003), xxix.

55. Pope Paul VI, quoted in *Papal Addresses*, xxix.

56. Ibid., xxx.

57. Pope Paul VI, "Address to the Plenary Session and to the Study Week on the Subject 'Brain and Conscious Experience,'" in *Papal Addresses*, 185.

58. White, in Renner, "White's Anatomy."

59. R. J. White et al., "Cephalic Exchange Transplantation in the Monkey," *Surgery* 70, no. 1 (July 1971): 135–39.

60. Monica Robins, "As MetroHealth Prepares to Break Ground on New Hospital,

Here's a Look Back at Its History," WKYC, April 12, 2019, https://www.wkyc
.com/article/news/as-metrohealth-prepares-to-break-ground-on-new-hospital
-heres-a-look-back-at-its-history/95-3924d492-e4dd-450a-a6cf-32ed68470df0.

61. Robert J. White et al., "Recovery of the Subhuman Primate After Deep Cerebral
Hypothermia and Prolonged Ischaemia," *Resuscitation* 2, no. 2 ( June 1973): 117–22.

62. Robert J. White, "Preservation of Cerebral Function During Circulatory Arrest
and Resuscitation: Hypothermic Protective Considerations," *Resuscitation* 1, no. 2
( July 1972): 107–112, IN5, 113–115.

63. Catherine Robert, "Animal Experimentation and Evolution," *The American Scholar*
40, no. 3 (Summer 1971): 497–503.

64. Ibid., 501.

65. Ibid.

66. Ibid., 498.

67. Ibid., 499.

68. Ibid., 500.

69. Ibid.

70. Jeremy Bentham, *An Introduction to the Principles of Morals and Legislation*, quoted in
Peter Singer, "All Animals Are Equal," *Philosophic Exchange* 1, no. 5 (Summer 1974).

71. Peter Singer, "All Animals Are Equal," in Tom Regan and Peter Singer, eds., *Animal Rights and Human Obligations* (Englewood Cliffs, NJ: Prentice Hall, 1976),
79–80.

72. Robert, "Animal Experimentation and Evolution," 497–503.

73. Robert White, "Antivivisection: The Reluctant Hydra," *The American Scholar* 40,
no. 3 (Summer 1971): 503–12.

74. Ibid., 507.

75. Ibid.

76. Ibid.

77. Ibid., 504.

78. Harvey Cushing, quoted in White, "Antivivisection," 504.

79. White, "Antivivisection," 504.

80. Ibid., 506.

81. Ibid., 507.

82. Ibid.

83. Howard Yonas, interview with the author, Cleveland Heights, Ohio, August 13,
2018.

84. Donald McRae, *Every Second Counts* (New York: Penguin, 2007), ebook.

85. Ibid.

86. Ibid.

87. Associated Press, "Edmund Stevens, 81, a Reporter in Moscow for 40 Years, Is Dead," *New York Times*, May 27, 1992.

88. Veatch, "Case Studies in Bioethics."

89. Schmeck, "Medicine."

90. Robert White, interview by Hans Vladimirsky and Konstantin Razin, "The Questionable and Unquestionable in Brain Transplant Problems," *Moscow News* 42 (1975): 11.

91. Reuters, "Head Transplant Next Step—Prof.," *Ottawa Journal*, July 7, 1972.

92. Reuters, "What's Next? Head Transplant," *Tennessean*, July 8, 1972.

93. Robert White, quoted in Peggy Rader, "Surgeon Views Brain of Humans as 'Inner Space,'" *Akron Beacon Journal*, July 31, 1977.

94. Ibid.

95. Audio transcribed from *MotherBoard*, "Interview with Robert White," *A Monkey Head Transplant*. Produced by David Feinberg, July 9, 2009.

96. Ibid., YouTube video, https://youtu.be/TGpmTf2kOc0.

97. White, quoted in Rader, "Surgeon Views Brain of Humans as 'Inner Space.'"

98. Reuters, "What's Next? Head Transplant."

## CHAPTER 7: THE HUMAN ANIMAL

1. Patricia White, interview, June 15, 2019.

2. Kleban, "A Devout Neurosurgeon Studies the Brain with Medically Dazzling, Morally Puzzling Head Transplants."

3. Ibid.

4. Robert White, letter.

5. Peter Carlson, "The Great Silver Spring Monkey Debate," *Washington Post*, February 24, 1991.

6. Ibid.

7. Ibid.

8. Ibid.

9. Tom Regan, "The Case for Animal Rights," in Tom Regan and Peter Singer, eds., *Animal Rights and Human Obligations* (Englewood Cliffs, NJ: Prentice Hall, 1976).

10. Richard Lyons, "Does Everyone on This Ark Have a First-Class Ticket?," *New York Times*, April 30, 1978.

11. Tom Regan, "Why Death Does Harm Animals," in *Animal Rights and Human Obligations*, 153–57.

12. Alex Pacheco with Anna Francione, "The Silver Spring Monkeys," in Peter Singer, ed., *In Defense of Animals* (New York: Basil Blackwell, 1985), 135–47.

13. Ibid.

14. A. N. Rowan, "The Silver Spring 17," *International Journal for the Study of Animal Problems* 3, no. 3 (1982): 219–27.

15. Carlson, "The Great Silver Spring Monkey Debate."

16. Ibid.

17. Ibid.

18. Pacheco with Francione, "The Silver Spring Monkeys," 135–47.

19. Carlson, "The Great Silver Spring Monkey Debate."

20. *The Use of Animals in Medical Research and Testing: Hearings Before the Subcommittee on Science, Research, and Technology of the Committee on Science and Technology*, US House of Representatives, 97th Cong., 1st Session, October 13, 14, 1981, no. 68 (Washington, DC: US Government Printing Office, 1982).

21. Carlson, "The Great Silver Spring Monkey Debate."

22. *The Use of Animals in Medical Research and Testing.*

23. Ibid., 13.

24. Taub, quoted in ibid.

25. Tori DeAngelis, "Going to Bat for Science," *Monitor on Psychology* 38, no. 7 ( July/August 2007): 20, https://www.apa.org/monitor/julaug07/tobat.

26. Ibid.

27. Ibid.

28. Quoted in ibid.

29. White, "Antivivisection: The Reluctant Hydra," 504.

30. Ibid., 507.

31. Robert J. White, "Animal Ethics?," *Hastings Center Report* 20, no. 6 (November–December 1990): 43.

32. Robert White, "Thoughts of a Brain Surgeon," *Reader's Digest*, September 1978.

33. Robert White, "Dr. Robert J. White: Years Later, Patient's Case Still on His Mind," *News-Herald* (Willoughby, Ohio), January 3, 2010.

34. Ibid.

35. John Hubbell, "The Medical Wonders of Dr. Robert White," *Reader's Digest*, February 1977.

36. Robert White, "An Interesting Case of a Juvenile Vascular Malfunction," *News-Herald* (Willoughby, Ohio), September 5, 2010.

37. Robert White, letter, March 23, 1989.

38. Y. Takaoka, N. Taslitz, and R. J. White, "The Vascular Split Brain in the Monkey," *Anatomical Record* 184, no. 3 (1976): 595.

39. Robert White, letter, June 30, 1982.

40. Robert White, letter, March 3, 1982.

41. Robert White, letter, June 30, 1982.

42. Ibid.

43. Robert White, letter, March 23, 1989.

44. Robert White, letter, August 11, 1983.

45. White, "An Interesting Case of Juvenile Vascular Malformation."

46. Robert White, letter, August 11, 1983.

47. Robert White, "The Facts About Animal Research," *Reader's Digest*, March 1988, 127–32.

48. Ibid., 129.

49. Ibid., 131.

50. Ibid.

51. Manjila et al., "From Hypothermia to Cephalosomatic Anastomoses," 20.

52. White, "The Facts About Animal Research."

53. Ibid., 130.

54. Ibid.

55. "Animal Rights Activists Rally at Reader's Digest Briefly," *The Morning Call*, July 19, 1988.

56. Ingrid Newkirk, phone interview with the author, November 19, 2019.

57. Ibid.

58. Ingrid Newkirk and Robert White, Debate, City Club Cleveland, February 10, 1989.

59. Newkirk interview, November 19, 2019.

60. Keith Mann, *From Dusk 'til Dawn: An Insider's View of the Growth of the Animal Liberation Movement* (London: Puppy Pincher Press, 2007), 497.

61. David Bennun, "Dr. Robert White," *Sunday Telegraph Magazine*, 2000, archived at https://www.bennun.biz/interviews/drwhite.html.

62. Ibid.

63. Ibid.

64. John Rinaldi, interview with author, Cleveland, Ohio.

65. Robert White, interview, "The Man Who Believes in Body Transplants," *Q.E.D.* (London: BBC Worldwide, 1989).

66. Ibid.

67. White, quoted in Bennun, "Dr. Robert White."

68. Ingrid Newkirk and Robert White, Debate, City Club Cleveland, February 10, 1989.

69. Ibid.

70. Ibid.

71. Ibid.

72. Ibid.

73. Ibid.

74. Newkirk interview, November 19, 2019.

75. Ibid.

76. Bennun, "Dr. Robert White."

77. Christian Jungblut, *Meinen Kopf auf deinen Hals; Die neuen Pläne des Dr. Frankenstein alias Robert White* (Stuttgart, Germany: Hirzel, 2001), 76.

78. Ibid.

79. Ibid.

80. Ibid., 79.

## CHAPTER 8: THE PERFECT PATIENT

1. Christian Jungblut, *Meinen Kopf auf deinen Hals; Die neuen Pläne des Dr. Frankenstein alias Robert White* (Stuttgart, Germany: Hirzel, 2001), 19.

2. Grant Segall, "Dr. Robert J. White, Famous Neurosurgeron and Ethicist, Dies at 84," *Cleveland Plain Dealer*, September 16, 2010, last modified January 12, 2019, https://www.cleveland.com/obituaries/2010/09/dr_robert_j_white_was_a_world-.html.

3. James Renner, "White's Anatomy," *Cleveland Free Times*, March 7, 2007.

4. Jungblut, *Meinen Kopf auf deinen Hals*, 185.

5. Ibid., 94.

6. Nicholas Regush, "Doctor Wants to Transplant Human Heads Soon," *Sightings*, Second Opinion, ABC News, June, 1, 2000.

7. Ibid.

8. Jungblut, *Meinen Kopf auf deinen Hals*, 94.

9. National Conference of Commissioners on Uniform State Law, "Uniform Determination of Death Act," 1981.

10. Ibid.

11. Jungblut, *Meinen Kopf auf deinen Hals*, 169.

12. Ibid, 168.

13. Ibid.

14. Ibid., 179.

15. Ibid., 67.

16. Ibid., 173.

17. Bennun, "Dr. Robert White."

18. Jungblut, *Meinen Kopf auf deinen Hals*, 21.

19. Bennun, "Dr. Robert White."

20. "Dynamic Coating & Craig Vetovitz," Channel 23 News, https://www.youtube.com/watch?v=9MnpMZ8-Av4.

21. Ibid.

22. Per Dr. J. P. Conomy, based upon his neurological evaluation of Craig Vetovitz in 1976, recounted here with the permission of Vetovitz's son Kreg Vetovitz.

23. "Your Head in His Hands," *Times Higher Education*, October 29, 1999.

24. Kreg Vetovitz, phone interview with author, October 29, 2019.

25. Sue Hively, "Couple's Plans Call for Two Homes in One," *Cleveland Plain Dealer*, January 13, 1979.

26. Ibid.

27. Josh Taylor, "Today's Profile," *Cleveland Plain Dealer*, July 16, 1991.

28. Alasdair Palmer, "Getting Tired of Your Body? Why Not Try a New One," *Sunday Telegraph/Edmonton Journal*, December 21, 1996.

29. Based on numbers of 2011; Kim Zuber and Jane S. Davis, "Kidney Transplantation: Who Is Eligible?," *Clinician Reviews* 21, no. 10 (October 2011): 19–23.

30. Ibid.

31. Putre, "The Frankenstein Factor."

32. Palmer, "Getting Tired of Your Body?"

33. Putre, "The Frankenstein Factor."

34. Ibid.

35. Ibid.

36. Ibid.

37. Kreg Vetovitz, phone interview with author, October 29, 2019.

38. Putre, "The Frankenstein Factor."

39. Ibid.

40. Jungblut, *Meinen Kopf auf deinen Hals*, 2.

41. Bennun, "Dr. Robert White."

42. Adapted from Jungblut, *Meinen Kopf auf deinen Hals*, 9–11.

43. Palmer, "Getting Tired of Your Body?"

44. Ibid., 132.

45. Glenn Zorpette and Carol Ezzell, "Your Bionic Future: As Life and Technology Merges, They Will Both Become More Interesting," *Scientific American* 10, no. 3 (Fall 1999): 4.

46. Ibid.

47. Ibid.

48. Ibid.

49. Ibid.

50. Ibid.

51. Ibid.

52. Ibid.

53. Ibid.

54. Ibid.

55. Jonathan Leake, "Surgeon Plans Head Transplant," *Sunday Times* (London), August 28, 1999.

56. U.S. Feature Syndicate Edit International and Taiwan News, "US Surgeon to Perform World's First Human-Head Transplant," *Tehran Times*, July 16, 2001.

57. Harold Hillman, "What Are the Prospects for Body Transplant?," *Ethical Record*, January 2000, 10.

58. Lou Jacobson, "A Mind Is a Terrible Thing to Waste," *Field Notes* (blog), *Lingua Franca*, 1997, http://linguafranca.mirror.theinfo.org/9708/fn.9708.html.

59. "Craig's Head to Be Moved to a New Body," NYHETERsön, July 8, 2001 (Swedish).

60. Kreg Vetovitz interview, October 29, 2019.

61. "Transplanted Heads," *Süddeutsche Zeitung*, August 25, 2000.

62. Ibid.

63. Ibid.

64. "A Little Off the Top," *Wired*, January 1, 2000.

65. Robert White, "Cleveland Visits Lenin's Brain," unpublished essay, White family archive.

66. Robert White, "A Halloween Tale: Where Is Lenin's Brain?," *News-Herald* (Willoughby, Ohio), October 25, 2009.

67. White, "Cleveland Visits Lenin's Brain."

68. Ajay Kamalakaran, "Nostalgia for the Russia of the 2000s," *Russia Beyond*, January 14, 2017.

69. Boris Fishman, "In Moscow, An Unexpected Creative Revolution," *Travel + Leisure*, October 28, 2015.

70. Michael White, email, July 12, 2019.

71. Jungblut, *Meinen Kopf auf deinen Hals*, 186.

72. "A Little off the Top."

73. Danielle Elliott, "Human Head Transplant Is 'Bad Science,' Says Neuroscientist," CBS News, July 2, 2013.

74. "Frankenstein Fears After Head Transplant," BBC News, April 6, 2001.

75. Bennun, "Dr. Robert White."

76. Ibid.

## CHAPTER 9: WHAT IF WE DON'T NEED THE SPINAL CORD?

1. "Reeve Ad Inspiring or Misleading?" CBS News, January 28, 2000.

2. David Ewing Duncan, "Biotech & Creativity: Quadriplegic Fitted with Brain Sensor Ushers in Cybernetic Age," *SFGate*, December 5, 2004.

3. Ibid.

4. Ibid.

5. M. D. Serruya et al., "Instant Neural Control of a Movement Signal," *Nature* 416, no. 6877 (March 14, 2002): 141–42.

6. Mary Beckman, "Monkey See, Cursor Do," *Science*, March 14, 2002.

7. Robert Lee Hotz, "Device Translates Brain's Energy into Actions: Nonsurgical Mind-Computer Link Could Assist Patients Unable to Move or Speak," *Los Angeles Times*, December 10, 2004.

8. Duncan, "Biotech & Creativity."

9. Sabin Russell, "Quadriplegic's Mind Able to Control Matter: Mind Reading a Success for Quadriplegic," *SFGate*, July 13, 2006.

10. Duncan, "Biotech & Creativity."

11. Ibid.

12. Russell, "Quadriplegic's Mind Able to Control Matter."

13. Robert White, "Future Wiring of Your Mind," *News-Herald* (Willoughby, Ohio), August 3, 2008.

14. Ibid.

15. Ibid.

16. Ibid.

17. Ibid.

18. Ibid.

19. Ibid.

20. Frank Spotnitz, interview with the author, July 20, 2018.

21. Ibid.

22. Ibid.

23. Ibid.

24. Ibid.

25. Frank Lovece, "The X-Files: I Want to Believe," film review, *Film Journal International*, July 24, 2008.

26. Roger Ebert, "The X-Files: I Want to Believe," film review, *Chicago Sun Times*, July 24, 2008.

27. Michael White, interview with author, Willoughby, Ohio, January 9, 2019.

28. Michael White, phone interview with author, August 13, 2019.

29. Patty White, letter, August 14, 2019.

30. Ibid.

31. Robert J. White, "You Learn a Lot About Yourself as a Patient," *News-Herald* (Willoughby, Ohio), June 7, 2009.

32. Ibid.

33. Joseph Murray, "Significance," Nobel Prize Nomination of Robert White, February 10, 2010.

34. Joseph Murray, email to Robert White, Friday, January 22, 2010, 10:16 a.m.

35. Joseph Murray, "History," Nobel Prize Nomination of Robert White, February 10, 2010.

36. Murray, "Significance."

37. Joseph Murray, email to Robert White, "Nobel Prize Nomination," Tuesday, January 12, 2010, 9:23 a.m.

38. Ibid.

39. Rachel Becker, "Spinal Implants Help Treat Paralysis but Aren't Ready for Primetime," *The Verge*, November 3, 2018.

40. Angus Chen, "Spinal Stimulator Implant Gives Paralytic Patients a Chance to Regain Movement," *Scientific American*, October 31, 2018.

41. Eliza Strickland, "Brain and Spine Implants Let a Paralyzed Monkey Walk Again: This First-in-Primate Study Tested Out Tech for Future Human Trials," *IEEE Spectrum*, November 10, 2016.

42. Ibid.

43. Brian Borton, quoted in Strickland, "Brain and Spine Implants."

44. Benedict Carey, "Once Paralyzed, Three Men Take Steps Again with Spinal Implant: An Experimental, Pacemaker-Like Device Offers Hope for Treating Spinal Injuries," *New York Times*, October 31, 2018.

45. Becker, "Spinal Implants Help Treat Paralysis."

46. Pallab Ghosh, "Spinal Implant Helps Three Paralysed Men Walk Again," BBC News, October 31, 2018.

47. Ibid.

48. Carey, "Once Paralyzed, Three Men Take Steps Again."

49. "Brain-computer Interface Enables Paralyzed Man to Walk: Proof-of-Concept Study Shows Possibilities for Mind-Controlled Technology," *Science Daily*, September 24, 2015.

50. Robert White, "The Two-Headed Russian Dog," *News-Herald* (Willoughby, Ohio), August 22, 2010.

51. Ibid.

52. Ibid.

53. Ibid.

54. Manjila et al., "From Hypothermia to Cephalosomatic Anastomoses," 14–25.

55. Ibid.

56. Ibid.

## CONCLUSION: DR. FRANKENSTEIN'S REPRISE

1. Putre, "The Frankenstein Factor."

2. Sergio Canavero, "HEAVEN: The Head Anastomosis Venture Project Outline for the First Human Head Transplantation with Spinal Linkage (GEMINI)," *Surgical Neurology International* 4 (Suppl. 1) (June 13, 2013): S335–42.

3. Sharon Kirkey, "Head Case," *National Post*, August 2019.

4. Ibid.

5. Ibid.

6. Harold Hillman, "Dr. Robert J. White," *Resuscitation* 83 (2012): 18–19.

7. Paula Gould, "Mice Regrow Damaged Spinal Cord," *Nature*, November 9, 2004.

8. Ibid.

9. "Purdue Research Offers Hope for Canine, Human Spinal Injuries," *Purdue University News*, December 3, 2004.

10. Ibid.

11. Sam Kean, "The Plan to Save a Life by Head Transplant," *The Atlantic*, September 2016.

12. Ibid.

13. The talk appeared in September 2015; TED flagged this talk.

14. Kirkey, "Head Case."

15. Kean, "The Plan to Save a Life by Head Transplant."

16. Ibid.

17. Ibid.

18. Ibid.

19. Yarin Steinbuch, "Disabled Man Changes Mind About Head Transplant," *New York Post*, December 18, 2018.

20. Sharon Kirkey, "First Man to Sign Up for Head Transplant Bows Out, but Surgeon Insists List of Volunteers Is Still 'Quite Long,'" *National Post*, April 9, 2019.

21. Kean, "The Plan to Save a Life by Head Transplant."

22. Haybitch Abersnatchy [pseud.], "Where the Body Ends and the Self Begins," *Futurism* (blog), *Vocal*, 2017, https://vocal.media/futurism/where-the-body-ends-and-the-self-begins.

23. Robert White, "Head Transplants," *Scientific American Presents: Your Bionic Future*, Fall 1999, 24.

24. Kim Hjelmgaard, "Xiaoping Ren and Sergio Canavero Claim Spinal Cord Progress," *USA Today*, March 27, 2019.

## Photo Credits

# Index

United States:
  in arms race with Soviet Union, 33–36, 41
  industrialization in, 11, 231
  in medical science race with Soviet Union,
    4–5, 36–37, 46, 57, 59, 93, 101–2
  nuclear weapons of, 34–35
  in space race with Soviet Union, 3, 40–42,
    46, 57–59
Unity Laboratory of Applied Neurobiology,
  249
University College London, 250
University Hospitals of Cleveland, 55, 179, 233
uranium, 35
urea, 13
urine, as by-product of kidney function, 10,
  13, 25–26
*USA Today*, 257
USDA, 168
Utah, University of, 223

Valley Forge General Hospital, 15
Van Allen, James, 42
Vatican, biomedical ethics commission of,
  171, 189
Vatican City, 143, 144
veins, 17, 38, 39, 64, 72, 75, 119, 122, 124, 206,
  209
  blood clots in, 204
  jugular, 212, 248
  ligation of, 173
  revascularization and, 97
  vertebral sinus, 122
  *see also* arteries; blood flow
Velyaminov, I. A., 94
Venn diagram, 196
ventilators, 5, 78, 121, 130
ventricles, 2
Verdura Riva Palacio, Javier, at BRL, 62, 65,
  70–74, 76, 79, 105, 110, 118, 122
vertebral arteries, 106, 248
vertebral sinus vein, 122

Vetovitz, Craig, 199
  accident and paralysis of, 199–201, 202,
    204, 240
  as candidate for human head transplant,
    202, 205–6, 211–12, 213, 214, 221, 240
  kidney failure of, 202, 221, 255
  NASA research grants to, 199, 201
Vetovitz, Kreg, 203, 205
Vetovitz, Susan, 201
*Vice*, 230
Vietnam War, 85
virtual reality, 211
Vishnevsky, Alexander, 42, 96
vivisection, 149–50
  *see also* animal rights
Vogt, Oskar, 90
Võ Nguyên Giáp, 103
Voronezh region, Ukraine, 37
Voronezh State University, 38

*Washington Post*, 139, 162, 169
Watson, James, 188, 236
*Week, The*, 249
Wertheimer, Pierre, 78, 131
Western Reserve University Medical School,
  55, 59
    RJW's teaching at, 56, 63
    *see also* Case Western Reserve University
West Virginia University, 56
*Where Good Ideas Come From* (Johnson), 54
White, Catherine, 18, 21
White, Chris, 48, 56, 151
White, Danny, 68
White, Jim, 18, 181
White, Marguerite, 117, 181
White, Michael, 56, 116, 233
White, Patricia (RJW's wife), 27, 48, 56, 60,
  68, 69, 82, 86, 110, 121, 159, 161, 181,
  182, 193, 233
White, Patty (RJW's daughter), 56, 229–30,
  238

## *About the Author*

**BRANDY SCHILLACE** (skil-AH-chay), PhD, works at the intersections of medicine, history, science, and literature. A one-time museum professional and university professor, Brandy is editor in chief of BMJ's *Medical Humanities* journal and runs the *MH* podcast on issues of social justice. Nonfiction includes *Death's Summer Coat: What the History of Death and Dying Teaches Us About Life and Living,* and *Clockwork Futures: The Science of Steampunk.* Dr. Schillace is a 2018 winner of the Arthur P. Sloan Science Foundation Award and has appeared on Travel Channel's *Mysteries at the Museum* and NPR's *Here and Now.* She has bylines at *Scientific American, Globe and Mail, HuffPo,* and *CrimeReads.*

Brandy grew up in an underground house next to a cemetery in abandoned coal land, had a pet raccoon, and still spends a lot of time in graveyards. Her research has taken her to catacombs, cholera cemeteries, research labs, and medical museums from New York to London, Oslo to Moscow. (She has also been in a lot of basements.)